Radiant Wise Woman

"Lee Sumner Irwin dispels the limiting messages women have been told for generations about what it means to get older. *Radiant Wise Woman*, an inspiring read, brings us to midlife wonder realizing that we have our best years yet to live."

—Kristine Carlson, *New York Times* best-selling author of Don't Sweat the Small Stuff books

"There has always been a stigma about menopause. Lee Sumner Irwin shatters the old beliefs and brings a refreshing new approach to thriving as your body changes through menopause. Every woman should read this book."

—Mal Duane, author of *Broken Open: Embracing Heartache & Betrayal as Gateways to Unconditional Love*

"I wish I'd had Lee Sumner Irwin's perspective when I was going through menopause. A generous wise woman, she has reframed this change as both an invitation and an initiation into an even more compelling stage of life. Her experience and guidance will help you transform drama and resistance into a new story of what's possible for your wisdom years."

—Gail Larsen, author of *Transformational Speaking: If You Want to Change the World, Tell a Better Story*

"In this book, Lee Sumner Irwin shares wisdom teachings to help menopausal and postmenopausal women reclaim joy, embrace abundance, and unlock their full potential. Even the practices feel like a warm hug that says, 'It's okay—allow yourself to soften, be feminine, be wonderful.' *Radiant Wise Woman* not only delivers a hopeful message for individual women but also provides a framework for collaborating collectively."

—Dr. Manja Podratz, founder of
the Collaborative Research Center for Consciousness Studies

"Lee Sumner Irwin's guidance for women going through perimenopause and menopause is refreshing, powerful, and incredibly supportive. Her wise words, reflections, and exercises lead women inward toward wholeness. We need more resources like this to remind women that menopause is a powerful initiation and a doorway to mature feminine wisdom."

—Cathy Skipper, author of *The Alchemy of Menopause:
The Journey of Stepping Into Our Power
and Becoming Who We Truly Are*

"*Radiant Wise Woman* is the bible for midlife transition I wish I'd had before being blindsided at age forty-five by full-blown menopause. Irwin covers every aspect of this potentially wonderful time of transformation if you're equipped with the knowledge, tools, and resources she provides. And who doesn't want to play Joygasm Bingo?"

—c.René Washington, author of *Take the Trip!
4 Journeys Every Midlife Woman Needs to Live in Purpose
and Freedom* and podcast host of *The Midlife Remix*

"In *Radiant Wise Woman*, Lee Sumner Irwin empowers women to celebrate and hone the wisdom of their bodies at a time usually associated with a loss of femininity. Insightful and reassuring, her book lights the way for women to shine their brightest at this often misunderstood season of their lives."

—Lanier Scott Isom, author of *Grace and Grit:
My Fight for Equal Pay and Fairness at Goodyear and Beyond*
with Lilly Ledbetter

Radiant Wise Woman

Breaking Free from the Myths of Menopause and Aging

LEE SUMNER IRWIN

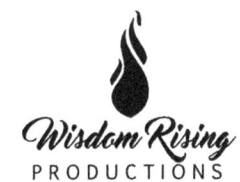

Wisdom Rising
PRODUCTIONS

Chapel Hill, North Carolina

Published by: Wisdom Rising Productions
1710 East Franklin Street #1053
Chapel Hill, NC 27514
www.radiantwisewoman.com

Editor: Ellen Kleiner
Cover design: Denise Sumner Bryant

First Edition

The contents of this book are for educational purposes only and not intended as a replacement for diagnosis or treatment of any physical, emotional, or medical condition. The reader should consult their health professional for treatment and make use of information in this book only as an adjunct to such treatment. In the event the reader uses information herein, the author and publisher shall assume no responsibility for any direct or indirect consequences.

Copyright © 2022 by Lee Sumner Irwin

All rights reserved. No part of this publication, except for brief quotations embodied in reviews or for other noncommercial uses permitted by copyright law, may be reproduced, stored in retrieval systems, distributed, or transmitted in any form or by any means—electronic, mechanical, photocopying, recording, or otherwise—without written permission of the publisher.

Printed in the United States of America

Publisher's Cataloging-in-Publication Data

Names: Irwin, Lee S., 1951- author.
Title: Radiant wise woman / Lee Sumner Irwin.
Description: First edition. | Chapel Hill, North Carolina : Wisdom Rising Productions, [2022] | Includes bibliographical references.
Identifiers: ISBN: 979-8-9850465-0-2 (paperback) | 979-8-9850465-1-9 (ebook) | LCCN: 2021920304
Subjects: LCSH: Aging–Psychological aspects. | Menopause–Psychological aspects Menopause–Health aspects. | Middle-aged women–Psychological aspects. | Middle-aged women–Health and hygiene. | Middle-aged women–Sexual behavior. | Older women–Psychological aspects. | Older women–Health and hygiene. | Older women–Sexual behavior. | Female orgasm. | Feminist spirituality. | Archetype (Psychology) | Self-realization in women. | Self-actualization (Psychology) | Self-acceptance in women.
Classification: LCC: HQ1206 .I79 2022 | DDC: 305.244/2–dc23

1 3 5 7 9 10 8 6 4 2

*For every woman who
bravely moves through the unknown
and for Vera, Kian, and the
generations to come*

In Gratitude…

I offer a deep bow of gratitude to everyone who helped birth this book, giving thanks for their gifts and the light and love they have shared.

Thank you to my inner Maiden, Queen, and Wise Woman, as well as the ancestors and guides who nudged me to write the first pages and connected me with helpers all along the way—I respect you and I love you. I am grateful to my Cherokee great-grandfather, Josef, who introduced me to my long line of female ancestors, medicine women who honored the stars, stones, rivers, and moon. I send love to the women in my family who nurtured me while they lived and are always with me in spirit: my mother Amy Bass Sumner, grandmother Ruby Lee Sumner, sister Camille Butler, guardian ancestor Fannie Davis, and Aunt Lillian, who was like a mother to me.

I am indebted to the many women I interviewed, for their willingness to share generously from their hearts and for their permission, in service to all women, to weave their stories with mine. I am humbled by my beloved clients who have trusted me with their deepest desires over the past twenty years. Special thanks to Deborah Boswell for her steadfast encouragement, Gerber daisies, and love.

I have been blessed by the guidance of numerous teachers and mentors. Thank you to Vassa Neimark, Dawn Lianna, Betsey Grady, Rosa Sepulveda, and Carol Fitzpatrick for revealing what lies beyond the physical dimension and lighting my path forward.

Kudos and gratitude to my publishing team extraordinaire, whose expertise and creative gifts brought this book into the world. To Ellen Kleiner of Blessingway Authors' Services, my boundless gratitude for her meticulous editing and patient, devoted guidance through every step of the publishing process. Love to my dear sister, Denise Bryant, who gave the priceless gifts of her personal support and brilliant creativity in the book cover and interior design.

The kinship of a writing community has been invaluable on this journey. I offer thanks to the Book Doulas, author Kristine Carlson, and editor Debra Evans—who set my feet firmly on the author's path—and to the writers in our circle: Sylvia Bento, Jesua Wight, Lisa Grafos, Liz McDonald, and Samantha Sweetwater. Thanks also to Gail Larsen, Theresa Thorne, Melanie Votaw, Lynn Duvall, Lanier Scott Isom, and Jane Trechsel for their candid feedback that helped shape a clear and compelling message.

I am grateful to friends and family members who believed in the potential of this book and whose love is infused in every page. For seeing me and hearing my desire to bring this book to life I offer thanks to Sue Varga, Tricia Acheatel, Elizabeth Wangler, Candace Pearl, Laurie Seymour, Andrea Luchese, Jennifer Schmidt, C. René Washington, Jasper Elliott Wolfe, Alexandra Ross, Lindsey Mullen, Margaret Pavela, Anne Ford, Vic Hale, Kathryn Barr, Sharon Cook, Nancy Jackson, Sean Hughes, Avanti Paul, Christa Irwin, and Tina Ogden.

I have been inspired by my Witchy Sisters—Dariana Dervis, Donna Matthews, and Jan Sharpe. Thank you for cheering me on, feeding me, and enticing me to come outside and play.

Blessings to the women in the Elevate group—Cheryl Blossom, Harsimrit Kaur Khalsa, Kimberly Adams, Christina Solstad, Simone Janssen, and my buddy coach Johanna McClain—for listening to my plans every month, keeping my feet on the ground, and helping me focus on my big "why." I send fond appreciation to the original Esther's Girls—Lyn Buchanan, Martha Hunter, Janet Raines, and Debbie Blackmon.

I offer my deep gratitude and love to Kent, my spouse and spiritual partner, who dares to be vulnerable, lifts me up when I stumble, and holds me in the highest light every step of the way.

Contents

Introduction: A New Map for Aging   1

1   **The Three Energies of Womanhood: The Maiden, Queen, and Wise Woman**   11
Inner Allies on Your Journey of Transformation

2   **Second Spring: Coping with the Shifts and Myths of Menopause**   31
Honoring Hormones, Body Changes, and Intuitive Insights

3   **Honey, Read This: For the Men**   55
Sharing Concerns about Menopause

4   **Flying Free on Wings of Forgiveness**   67
Releasing Destructive Patterns and Old Hurts

5   **Chaos to Calm**   81
Letting Your Wounds Become Your Wisdom

6   **Embracing the Wildness Within**   91
Reconnecting with Nature and the Sacred Power of Your Body and Voice

7   **Joygasms Galore**   107
Feeling More Sensual, Sexy, and Happy

8	**Attracting an Angel Posse** *The Transformative Power of Friendship, Community, and Creative Collaboration*	127
9	**Imagining a New Story of Aging** *Crafting and Living Your Legacy*	143
10	**Awakening to Your Divine Blueprint** *Realizing Your Radiance*	157

Resources	167
Notes	175
Bibliography	181

INTRODUCTION

A New Map for Aging

The future is completely open, and we are writing it moment to moment.

~Pema Chödrön

As their birthday cakes fill up with candles, women at age forty or better often start to believe the myth that the best years of their lives are over. They might worry that their minds aren't as sharp as they once were or that their energy, attractiveness, and sexy mojo are fading. They may think they're going to wither up and die because their childbearing days have passed or that they're losing the essence of who they were.

You have had a full life, yet you may also have an inner sense that something is missing and wonder what could fill the void. Or you may see your life as sand passing through an hourglass, with most of the sand in the bottom part, and think, "It's time to slow down and get in my rocking chair."

But what if you decide not to accept these limiting ideas? What if you could instead feel like my friend Nancy, who is living life to the fullest and insists: "At the end of my life, I don't want to be carried across the finish line feet first. I want to come careening across it on a Boogie Board with my arms raised to the sky, squealing, 'Whee!'" What if you believe you are actually in the wisdom years of your life, imbued with the immense potential this phase offers, such as the ability to:

Introduction

- Learn to truly love yourself
- Enjoy more laughter, connection, and wonder, free from past traumas
- Attract people who open you to more love and pleasure
- Access three types of inner female energy—the Maiden, Queen, and Wise Woman—to support your creativity and growth
- Discover your unique gifts and offer them to the world as a legacy
- Feel more alive, moving through each day with joy and grace

Viewing postmenopause as the time for developing these abilities turns the hourglass upside down, presenting the future as brimming with possibilities for new insights, greater wisdom, and more meaningful personal accomplishments.

Here's the truth: In the Western world, there's been no true map for aging, but now it's becoming ever clearer that devastating messages of limitation imposed on generations of women about what it means to get older are simply wrong. Based on my interviews and conversations with women entering their wisdom years, I've found that after menopause the potential to experience sexual enjoyment, happiness, and self-understanding is greater than ever before.

In Chinese medicine, the menopausal years are known as a woman's second spring.[1] This is the time when life energy is directed inward instead of outward. In the childbearing and menstrual years, energy goes to the pelvic area; during menopause, energy shifts to the heart.[2] From this place, you can

Introduction

learn to speak your truth, find your deepest life purpose, and give expression to it. In this state, past wounds become your wisdom, with new insights leading to the release of shame and pain you may have carried for decades, so you can finally break free from unhealthy patterns and confusion to enjoy a life of well-being. In other words, the feeling that you're being turned inside out as you transition into menopause actually signals the potential for a stirring rebirth, with the opportunity to not merely write a new chapter of your life but compose a whole new book. That new life is yours when you begin to pay attention to the ancient wisdom hidden within your body, trust your intuitive promptings, and act on your hard-won understanding.

Instead of viewing the menopausal and postmenopausal years as a time of diminishing possibilities, to cultivate a new perspective on aging the real questions to ask yourself are: What expectations and hopes do I have for my second spring? Am I willing to open myself to an expanded life of joy, wonder, and fulfillment beyond what I experienced when I was younger, further enriching my life and increasing my awareness of its value and meaning?

This book is about the prospects of creating an even more engaging life after menopause. It was conceived while facing questions about my own potential as I grew older. When a psychic friend told me I would start writing a book within six months, I scoffed at her. But one day a few months later, as I settled into my desk chair and sipped my morning tea, I felt a subtle urge to open my computer and start typing. My conscious mind switched off while my fingers flew across the keyboard documenting the ideas that surged into my mind. Two hours later, slightly dizzy as if emerging from a trance,

I stared in disbelief at eleven pages of writing. In meditation the next morning, I saw a vision of a woman with straight black hair, wearing a vibrant red dress and silver-tooled belt and carrying a basket overflowing with corn—a strong indigenous woman embodying qualities of the divine feminine. She told me: "Speak to the women's hearts. Surrender to the flow." Over the next three years, despite doubt and "labor pains," I did my best to follow her counsel in birthing this book to guide women through the transition of menopause and aging.

During twenty years as a transformational coach for hundreds of women around the world, in-depth interviews with women of all ages, and intimate conversations with friends, as well as my own experiences, I have tracked the recurring patterns many of us face as we navigate the choppy waters of aging. I've talked with women who, even in their late thirties, are anxious about getting older and secretly grieving over what they think they must give up. They tell themselves, "I'm not ready for this. Will I have to change how I dress and act? I haven't accomplished the things I wanted to. Do I have to give up on the dreams I've had? It feels like I'm running out of time and the doors of opportunity are closing. Have I missed the boat?"[3]

The two decades of my own life between college and my forties were filled with difficult, burning questions: What am I supposed to be doing? Should I stay in this relationship or not? What is my purpose for being on the planet? Then in my late forties, as life suddenly came to resemble a tilt-a-whirl ride, the predominant question was: What is going on with my body? I was embarking on perimenopause, which was like puberty gone haywire, with similar hormonal challenges but

Introduction

different symptoms. Things were about to get even crazier as I encountered the maze of menopause before landing on my feet in the third phase of womanhood—the wisdom years—when I've felt more alive, healthy, and happy than ever before because I finally know who I am and what I'm here to do.

As women, we go through big changes in midlife—in our bodies, in our relationships and families, and in our feelings and perceptions about ourselves—without effective guidance. The changes we face are as dramatic as those in earlier phases of life that altered us, such as learning to walk, leaving home to live on our own, becoming a mother, or starting a career, but rarely are these changes addressed. To maintain a healthy perspective and use age-related fluctuations to our advantage, women need to talk about the implications of such changes and how to deepen our understanding of not only the challenges of aging but also its potential benefits. Unfortunately, few doctors have the time or training to walk us through this phase of life. Most of our mothers didn't teach us about it or even acknowledge their own fears and discomforts around it, ensuring that the story about growing older remained ominous and limiting, shrouded by a collective anxiety.

In the past, women's roles in society were assigned, and most conformed to these expectations, which offered women a sense of security. Women today are freeing themselves from the trap of an unexamined life, questioning the old rules and stereotypes of womanhood and insisting on greater self-determination and self-fulfillment. And while the genie has been out of the bottle since the cultural revolution of the 1960s and 1970s, society's perception of older women has not kept pace with these breakthroughs. Recently I asked Siri, the assistant on my smart phone, "What is the definition of crone?" She had the audacity to respond, in a cheerful voice, "Crone means an old woman who is thin and ugly." Clearly we have a long way to go to fully understand the ongoing false perceptions about female aging and their effects on women's potential. Toward that end, we need to have candid conversations with one another, bringing our concerns, experiences, questions, and epiphanies to light. We need to know that what we're going through is not an end but a beginning, a natural progression to our wisdom years. Fortunately, women on the journey of self-discovery are now rethinking life's stages in novel and more expansive ways. Changing the prevailing story of aging, too often depicted as unpleasant, to an innovative and rewarding adventure is the ultimate mission of this book.

Think of this volume as your "pillow book," to be kept at your bedside for enjoyment and support. Traditionally, pillow books were written by women in tenth-century Japanese court society to convey their private thoughts and feelings to other women and, often embellished with erotic images and teachings, were intended as guides to sexual practices.[4] The insights offered in this book, based on the experiences of many women who have lived through the often challenging transition from the menopausal years to the wisdom years, likewise provide a road map to a vibrant new life, with U-turns, roadblocks, and signposts clearly marked. Discussions in the chapters that follow address some of the most important aspects of your life—health, emotional well-being, friendship, spiritual growth, and freedom from past pain. Revealing stories illuminate the benefits of receiving, forgiving others and yourself, and getting excited about what's next on your journey. You will come to know that your years in menopause and beyond are not a time of decline but instead represent

Introduction

the full flowering of your true essence. You will feel yourself acclimating to limitlessness. You will sense your enthusiasm rekindling and will gain a new appreciation of yourself—feeling welcomed, loved, and worthy. You will know that you are a vital expression of divine potential. As a result, you will likely see meaningful changes in your life. You may begin dusting off an old dream, change careers, open a business, stand up for a cause you believe in, move to a new home, or welcome in new love.

Although these big changes can feel like the ground beneath you is shifting, they can also open up new sources of support and guidance. For instance, you're likely to meet women who have gone through similar struggles and emerged as inspiring role models. You will easily recognize them by the transformations they describe and the light in their eyes. In the words of a client in her early fifties reflecting on the impact of changes she underwent during our coaching partnership the previous year: "I can feel these deep changes in how I approach life. I'm doing a lot less striving and proving, and so much more enjoying and savoring. I have more time for myself because saying no is getting easier. I am no longer scared of this unknown space I'm entering. Instead, I'm curious and excited about what is next for me. I realize I've waited my whole life to finally feel comfortable in my body. So I can now watch this process with curiosity and wonder, trusting my intuition to guide me to the next right thing."

This book may be read either alone at your own pace or with a small group in which each person speaks candidly, without shame or hiding behind a mask of perfection. In letting facades fall and illusions slough away, we come into alignment with our luminous essence and encounter our own radiance.

Introduction

To derive the greatest benefit from your reading experience, set powerful intentions—plans to commit yourself to specific courses of action—along the way. Doing so can help you integrate new information into your awareness and bring its key points to life in your day-to-day actions, thus shaping the outcomes you will eventually experience. One possibility would be to create intentions based on the practices at the end of each chapter. In this case, upon completing each practice you would jot down the relevant attitudes and behaviors you plan to cultivate and when you will set them in motion. You might write, for instance:

I will tune in to the supportive energies of my inner Maiden, Queen, and Wise Woman today.

Each week I will deal with at least one issue that is zapping my energy.

This weekend I will set aside two hours to enjoy connecting with my senses while walking in nature.

Starting tomorrow, I intend to forgive people from my past who have hurt me.

From this point forward, I will be a better friend to myself.

To help manifest your desires, read the statements aloud; decorate them with a colored pen; or paint, dance, or sing them. Activating your intentions in this way will ease you into adopting the attitude needed to fulfill them and ultimately awaken your greatest potential.

It's time to say yes to the Radiant Wise Woman within as you move into your wisdom years. She patiently awaits your

Introduction

willingness to find her and bring her forth. May you delight in each moment you spend traveling the bright path of renewal and giving birth to your wild, orgasmic, and resplendent self.

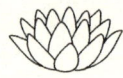

*And you? When will you begin that
long journey into yourself?*

~Rumi

CHAPTER 1

The Three Energies of Womanhood: The Maiden, Queen, and Wise Woman

Inner Allies on Your Journey of Transformation

In the 1830s, over sixteen thousand Cherokee people were forcibly removed from their ancestral homelands in the lush, green southern United States to trek 2,200 miles to the dry, desolate reservations in Oklahoma over what is known in Cherokee as Nunna daul Tsuny, "The Trail Where They Cried," where more than four thousand died.[1] One winter evening as the families were marched west along John's Creek in northern Alabama, they felt ice crunch under their feet and, clutching their thin blankets close to their bodies, heard an owl in the treetops hooting a warning. When the soldiers ordered that there would be no tents erected that night for shelter, the grandmothers, considered the wise elders of their clans who were revered and consulted on tribal matters, huddled with the children in a circle on the frozen ground, wrapping their bodies around their beloved young ones. The next morning all the grandmothers were dead but all the children had survived.[2]

Imagine what the world would look like if we emulated those Cherokee grandmothers, tapping into that tender yet fierce love as we speak truth to power, stand up to misogyny and lies, decry the exploitation of children, and say "no more" to the destruction of our natural world.

Such courage, love, and wisdom expressed with grandeur and generosity beyond logic reflect the archetype of the Wise Woman, one of three powerful female energies existing within us as allies to help us sustain life for future generations by altering our views of aging and shifting old paradigms of power, greed, and separation. Of these three inner allies, the first is the Maiden, characterized by sensuality and creativity. The second is the Queen, noted for strength and nurturing. And the third is the Wise Woman, demonstrating gifts of intuition, boldness, and grace.

Although we can access all three of these female energies at any time during our adult life, their characteristics correspond closely with particular phases of womanhood. We are most affected by the Maiden part of us in our twenties and early thirties, the Queen aspect from our mid-thirties to menopause, and the Wise Woman aspect during our post-menopausal years. Yet to be fully who we are and change the world for the better, we need to be aware of all of them and invite them to guide us throughout our life journey. So let's explore each of these archetypes.

The Maiden is innocent and vulnerable. She relies on her gut feelings and embraces life with a childlike sense of wonder. She's creative, playful, and free. She's in touch with sensual and sexual pleasure. She believes anything is possible, and she loves to manifest things quickly.

The Queen is clear, strong, and grounded. She nurtures herself and her female friendships and also provides a safe harbor for her family, her business, and her intimate relationships. She stands in her power, gets the help she needs, and

The Three Energies of Womanhood

sets healthy boundaries. She commands respect, not aggressively but with a serene, confident demeanor. The Wise Woman knows who she is and what she's meant to do. She relies on her well-honed intuition and sees beyond surface appearances. She isn't afraid to speak her truth and doesn't concern herself with what others think of her. As a result, she's often very straightforward. She actively contributes her gifts and leaves a legacy for generations to come. If there has been such a woman in your life who modeled courage, love, and generosity, you have likely found her inspirational. For me, it was the housekeeper I called Aunt Lillian, who cared for me every weekday when I was four and had a big, soft bosom for me to nestle into when I got scared. Closing my eyes, I can still taste the warm banana bread she baked for me, crumbly and fragrant with cinnamon. She would stop ironing my father's shirts and clap her hands in delight when I twirled around the living room, exclaiming, "That's my girl!" Her love and encouragement has remained with me, guiding me through six decades.

It is important to nurture and stay connected with all three of these energies of womanhood. It is equally essential to recognize the benefits that arise when they work together to maximize women's potential for creativity, growth, and happiness.

The Importance of Nurturing All Three Energies of Womanhood

When we are disconnected from the three female energies, unaware of how to access them or how they can work in tandem for our benefit, the consequences can be painful. For example, when the Maiden is not honored, a woman can become self-centered, focused on fulfilling her superficial desires, promiscuous, or afraid to give up control and open her heart to a partner.

When the Queen is not nurtured, her shadow side can emerge, causing a woman to abandon her feminine nature; use others to gain personal fame, money, and attention; neglect self-care; or take pride in the pressure she's under. She might develop a codependent relationship with her children or spouse, always catering to their demands over her own. Or she might start feeling chronically unfulfilled yet confused about how to improve her life.

When the Wise Woman is ignored, a woman's voice can become silenced and she can become afraid to remember who she is at her core, fearful that she'll be seen as too intense or quirky. Or she may smother her power, isolate herself, or become lethargic and depressed.

I've experienced many of these effects throughout my life. When I was ten years old, my mother took me to see the musical *Annie Get Your Gun*, which left an indelible impression on my vision of personal freedom. For months afterward, dressed in my boots, cowgirl hat, and brandishing two silver cap guns, I ran around the backyard singing "Don't Fence Me In," a song that became my inner anthem as I struggled against the constraints of life in the southern United States, where girls were trained to look pretty and be quiet. In my twenties and thirties, I didn't feel independent as a woman, didn't respect my own thinking, and was clueless when anyone asked me what I wanted, allowing myself to be treated like a doormat without realizing I was giving away my power. Clarissa Pinkola Estés's classic book *Women Who Run with the Wolves* articulates the impact of having only a certain restrained temperament and appearance be acceptable: "When women are relegated to

The Three Energies of Womanhood

moods, mannerisms, and contours that conform to a single ideal of beauty and behavior, they are captured in both body and soul, and are no longer free."[3]

In my late forties, while I traveled extensively as the owner of a thriving business, parented an active teenager, chronically argued with my boyfriend, and weathered the confusing symptoms of perimenopause, my inner voice geared up for a primal scream. I went through a series of mishaps. First, my car caught fire. A week later at work, I injured my back so badly I couldn't walk for a month. I was forced to lie still in bed as my mind reeled. Amidst the isolation of those weeks my intuition came to the rescue. Listening to it, I moved toward making some major changes, recalling the adage: "Why not go out on a limb? That's where all the fruit is." Over the next six months, I ended the ill-fated relationship with my boyfriend and left my career as an occupational therapist, despite having no job prospects and only a small nest egg to tide me over for a few months.

Taking these risks opened the door to new beginnings I never could have predicted. I moved back to my hometown and, through a series of synchronicities, discovered the profession of life coaching, meaningful work I felt I had been born to do. One day shortly after my move, a new friend invited me to come to the yoga class she was teaching. As I walked into her studio, I saw an attractive man standing at the door with a yoga mat tucked under his arm. I had the strange sensation of a fist hitting the center of my chest, and I heard a message in my head: "You're going to have a significant relationship with him." Initially the idea scared me silly, but gradually, over a two-year period, our friendship grew. Today, fifteen-plus years of marriage later, he has become my "S.P."—the spiritual partner and soul mate I had given up on ever having.

Reflecting on my years since menopause, I see that I have reconnected with the three female energies I hadn't even known existed in me. Now I not only have access to the Maiden, Queen, and Wise Woman but better understand how they can work together for my benefit. As a result, I wake up feeling excited about each new day. I have plenty of energy for things that matter to me. I know how to tap into my intuition, and I trust it over the directives of so-called experts and self-proclaimed gurus. My voice has awakened, and I speak my truth and sing in public (even if it's slightly off-key at times). I give myself permission to play and savor the small pleasures in each day. I've stopped hiding, which allows me to "go bigger" and pursue my life purpose with grace and ease. I now know that the challenges I faced in the past and the integration of the three feminine archetypes led me to my most fulfilling relationship, my new career, and better health, resulting in a joyful life beyond what I ever imagined.

You have likely weathered your own changes and losses. You may have said good-bye to loved ones, gotten divorced or fired, or given up on creative ambitions. Perhaps you stifled your playful self in service to a demanding job or children. You may have resigned yourself to an ever-smaller circle of people and experiences. You may have lost stamina, resilience, or suffered health challenges, and believe things will only go downhill from here. But learning how to access and integrate the three feminine archetypes can help make clear that what lies ahead may be the most exciting time in your life. The stories that follow show how these three energies mark stages in our lives and are also present throughout our lives; why their integration is important; and how you can access them to guide you in drawing on your innate strengths and gifts for greater fulfillment in life. They also illustrate how other women can help you tap into these three energies to maintain health and happiness and ultimately experience the fullness of womanhood.

The Wise Woman Needs the Maiden

While the Maiden is most commonly associated with sensuality and sexuality, a surprising truth is that women in the Wise Woman phase of life can reach their sexual peak when their Maiden self is also accessed. To comprehend how aspects of the Wise Woman interact with those of the Maiden, consider what happened to a sixty-year-old in her Wise Woman years who had lost connection with the Maiden self of her twenties.

Margie, a former coaching client who was single and recently retired from a demanding job as an executive at a large hospital, thought retirement would give her time to follow her creative impulses, but her sketchbooks and colored pencils were stuffed into boxes, and, when looking out at the flower garden she had envisioned, she saw only a few dried sunflowers. It seemed her life had become filled with only mundane activities such as making grocery lists, paying bills, and napping. Even her cat was lethargic. In truth, Margie was bored. Somewhere deep inside, the Maiden part of herself was eager to come out and engage with the world, but Margie had lost touch with that childlike aspect and, since retiring, had settled for a comfortable yet dull life.

One day when she received a message on social media from a man she had dated in college, her heart did a backflip. Margie agonized over whether to answer his message, but her Maiden self was nudging her, so she decided to reply to him. Choosing the path of fun and adventure, she and her former flame continued connecting online, catching up on where life had taken them—children grown and launched, divorces, careers, successes, and failures. They lived in different regions of the country, but over the next few months they decided to meet midway to explore their renewed friendship.

Happily, Margie found that the chemistry between them had not diminished, in spite of the man's thinning hair and her bad knees. Surprised to find that her desire for sex was even stronger than when she was young, she opened herself to new heights of pleasure that surpassed her former sexual encounters with him. "Now that I'm older it's easier to let go and enjoy myself in bed! He loves to see me happy, and I'm cherishing his attention," she said. Soon Margie also began restoring her garden to a lush oasis and sketching the flowers, which inspired her to sign up for a class in watercolor painting. After accessing her Maiden self, she experienced an infinitely richer life, and she is now a voluptuous Wise Woman who sees with the Maiden's eyes of wonder and possibility.

The Maiden Needs the Queen

We can call on the Queen, regardless of our stage in life, when insight and incisive action are needed to help us make a leap to a new path. The Queen asks us to welcome support and ultimately nurture others in return, as reflected in the following story.

Carole was a bright, funny, thoughtful friend in her late twenties, typically the years of the Maiden phase of womanhood. She was a survivor of childhood sexual abuse but had never dealt with the repercussions of that early violation of her innocence. In high school, she fell in love with a young man. She longed for his attention and approval, and over

The Three Energies of Womanhood

the next seven years devoted herself to giving him whatever she thought he wanted, unaware that she was suppressing her own desires. When he ignored her or betrayed her trust, instead of expressing how hurt she felt, she stifled her emotions. She had a few twenty-something girlfriends but was uncomfortable being the center of attention. So, instead of asking them for help, she listened to their problems. Disconnecting from the feelings in her body kept her cut off from her Maiden energy.

Fortunately, she had a supervisor at work who became an empathetic mentor. Sherry, in her mid-forties, strode confidently down the hall at work with her shoulders back and her head held high. She was perceptive and grounded, connected to her Queen energy, and she had a reputation around the office for being a steel fist in a velvet glove. One day Carole confided in Sherry, resulting in a dialogue that revealed a path forward where Carole could access her Queen self by trusting in the help offered by an older woman.

CAROLE: I'm so frustrated with my boyfriend. He tells me what to do and then criticizes me for being too "mousy." I keep trying hard yet feel like I can't win with him. I wish I knew what to do; whatever I try is the wrong thing. I feel so confused.

SHERRY: You know, we all need help sometimes. I remember feeling the same way when I was younger.

CAROLE: But you seem so sure of yourself, like you've got it all together.

SHERRY: Well, I made some big mistakes and fell flat on my face more than once. I learned a lot—mostly that I needed to ask for help. Thank goodness I met some amazing women who took me under their wings and believed in me until I could see my own strengths. I want you to know I'm here for you if you ever need a confidante.

CAROLE: Really? I wish I knew what to do about my boyfriend. He told me last week he wants to have an open relationship so that we can have sex with other people. I feel like I have to agree to let him have what he wants or he'll leave me and find someone else. But I know if I say yes I'll be seething inside. I get jealous when he even looks at another woman on the street.

SHERRY: I see how hard you're trying to make this relationship work. I wonder what your body is telling you. If your stomach could talk, what do you think it would say to you?

CAROLE: It feels like it's saying, "No way."

SHERRY: I can't tell you what the right choice is for you. That's your decision to make. But one important skill I've learned over the years is to listen to my gut. There's nothing wrong with you. We all get confused, and it's especially hard to give ourselves loving acceptance if we've been taught to be people-pleasers.

The Three Energies of Womanhood

Over the next year, Carole began to see herself as Sherry saw her—competent and worthy of respect. She did try the open relationship arrangement with her boyfriend, but it never felt right. So she eventually broke up with him and chose a new life path, going back to college to pursue her passion for graphic design. Carole had needed her Queen self to help her speak up, set healthy boundaries, and get a more balanced perspective on her gifts while pursuing her ambitions.

The Queen Needs the Wise Woman

The wise woman invites us to release past pain and embrace our intuition and true essence, as evidenced by the following story. Susie was forty-five, in the Queen phase of womanhood, when diagnosed with breast cancer. She was a fighter, both psychologically and literally—as a champion boxer and highly successful sales director in the competitive pharmaceutical industry. Her mother had recently died from breast cancer, so when Susie's doctor recommended that she undergo a mastectomy, chemotherapy, and radiation, she quickly agreed. Her Queen self, who knew how to get support, helped her take time off from her busy job to focus on self-care and accept help from her women friends. When she was too weak to get off the couch during chemo, they put healthy meals in a cooler outside her door each day, often with a funny card or an encouraging note.

Five years later Susie's physical scars were healed and she felt healthy, but while waiting for the results of a PET scan she was afraid the cancer had returned. When the letter from the lab finally arrived, her hands trembled so violently that she had trouble opening the envelope to read the terse report stating that she was cancer-free. After receiving the good news, Susie was surprised at how irritable she still felt, sniping at her colleagues and friends. She soon realized what was gnawing at her—a concern that even though she had been pronounced "clean" she needed to heal on an emotional level, suspecting that she had to face the pain of losing her mother.

As much as Susie longed for this deeper healing, she was afraid to dive in, and so she sought the energy and perspective of the Wise Woman for support. She found it reflected in a gifted professional bodyworker around her mother's age who eventually had, with therapeutic massage, helped Susie trace her sensations and emotions to the location in her body where she had first felt the disempowerment and illness. Breathing into the knots where her grief was stored, Susie was able to release the trauma, helping her complete a heroic journey from breakdown to breakthrough. A few months later she decided to follow her intuition and leave her all-consuming job to relocate to a less expensive part of the country closer to her son. She ultimately soared free, landing a part-time job with a nonprofit organization serving at-risk girls that helped her feel she was contributing to something greater than herself. Susie came to understand that due to the emotional and physical healing journey she had braved, she was now better equipped to guide young women she encountered through her work. And her younger sister and nieces told her they saw her as a model of the resilient older women they could one day become.

These three aspects of ourselves—the Maiden, Queen, and Wise Woman—each mark a predictable stage in womanhood, but they always need each other and thus require integration. The Maiden reminds us to stay connected to our imagination and sensual nature, to be playful and full of wonder. The Queen asks us to welcome support as we nurture others. The Wise Woman invites us to release the past and embrace our intuition and courage. Interwoven and always enlivening one another, these inner allies stand ready to help any time we feel weak or confused. Their love is endless, offering the support and clarity necessary for us to heal and improve our lives.

BREATHING SPACE

I'm eager to befriend my inner
Maiden, Queen, and Wise Woman.

I am grateful for the women
in my life who have guided me.

PRACTICE

How Well Are You Supported by the Maiden, Queen, and Wise Woman?

A simple way to assess how well you are supported by the three energies of womanhood involves three steps. First, select the phase you are currently in based on your age and stage of life:

Maiden: Twenties to early thirties
Queen: Mid-thirties to menopause
Wise Woman: Postmenopause

Next, familiarize yourself with the gifts of each phase, summarized as follows:

Maiden: Vulnerable, creative, and playful. She relies on her gut feelings and embraces life with a childlike sense of wonder. She is in touch with her sensuality and pleasure. She believes anything is possible and loves to manifest things quickly.

Queen: Clear, strong, and grounded. She nurtures herself as well as her female friendships and provides a safe harbor for her family, her business, and her intimate relationships. She stands in her power, gets the help she needs, and sets healthy boundaries. She commands respect, not aggressively but often with a serene demeanor.

Wise woman: Intuitive, feisty, and courageous. She knows who she is and what she's meant to do. Emotionally and spiritually mature, she sees beyond surface appearances. She's straightforward and not concerned with what others think of her. She actively contributes her gifts and leaves a legacy for generations to come.

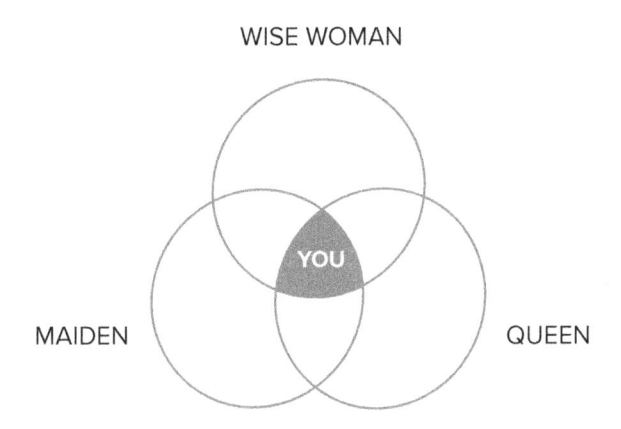

WISE WOMAN

MAIDEN   YOU   QUEEN

Finally, read the following three statements and write their corresponding number—1, 2, or 3—in the relevant circles above, labeled: Maiden, Queen, and Wise Woman.

1. *I wonder what happened to this part of myself. I've been unaware of it, ignored it, or abandoned it.*
2. *I sometimes feel connected to this aspect, but I know I don't have all her gifts.*
3. *I have easy access to this part of myself. She is fully integrated into my life. I listen to her guidance and feel supported by her.*

Now add up the numbers in the circles. If your total is between four and eight, you have enjoyed at least some of the gifts of these three allies. Invite all of them to further guide you as you break free from the myths of menopause and aging to reclaim your most vibrant self.

PRACTICE

Your Ideal Life—See It, Feel It, and Believe It

This practice helps you gain clarity about the look and feel of your ideal life so you will know the decisions that can help you achieve it.

1. Find a quiet place, either indoors or outdoors, surrounded by natural beauty.

2. With a journal and a colored pen at hand to record your thoughts, sit on a chair, a cushion, a rock, or the earth and take three deep breaths or enter a meditative state.

3. With a relaxed mind, ask yourself the following questions about your ideal life:

   Where am I?
   What am I doing?
   Who am I with?
   What delights me?
   What am I wearing?
   What do I see, hear, and smell?
   What am I looking forward to?
   How do I feel as all this is happening?

4. Spontaneously write down the thoughts that come to you, without worrying about your wording.

5. Feel your ideal life as if it were already happening. In the quantum field, it already is happening, and feeling this helps unlock the door to infinite possibilities.

6. Grab your phone, open a voice memo, and record your answers to the questions in #3.

7. Every night before going to bed, pop in your earbuds and listen to the recording you made about your ideal life.

This practice rewires your brain by opening up new neural pathways. The more you draw on the images and feelings you've tapped into, the more quickly your choices will bring you into your ideal life.

PRACTICE

The Radiance Menu

Each morning select from the following menu the options that most inspire you, then incorporate them into your day.

Body
- Drink a smoothie of fiber, protein, and healthy fat (such as coconut oil, avocado, or nut butter).
- Practice gentle stretches or bone-strengthening yoga poses.
- Dance to music that helps you connect with your body for 10 to 15 minutes.
- Eat plant-based foods mindfully, until you feel nourished but not stuffed.
- Tone your body with cardio and muscle-strengthening exercises for 30 minutes. Do this three times per week.

- Enjoy one or more orgasms, solo or with your partner.
- Take a luxurious bath of Epsom salts, essential oil, and coconut oil.
- Get bodywork or energy healing. Do this twice a month for stress relief and energetic balance.

Mind
- Read a page from an inspiring book.
- Choose an oracle card for guidance.
- Plug into a brainwave entrainment audio with earbuds to boost focus and creativity.
- Enjoy heart-connecting conversations with your partner, friends, or strangers.
- Before bedtime, listen to your recording of the ideal life you envision.

Spirit
- Say a wake-up prayer, such as: "Thank you for this day. Thank you for this life. Thank you for this body. Thank you for my loved ones and my ancestors. Thank you for my Maiden, Queen, and Wise Woman. Thank you for the beauty and meaning in my life. Thank you for helping me surrender more so I can serve more and love more." Then jump out of bed, raise your arms, and say: "Something amazingly awesome is coming to me today!"
- Meditate for at least 5 minutes.
- Immerse yourself in uplifting sounds; consider crystal bowls, birdsong, chanting, or Solfeggio frequencies.
- Dive into random acts of creation; dabble in a fun activity; get messy; marvel at colors or sounds.

The Three Energies of Womanhood

- Commune with nature: plants, water, wind, trees, pets.
- Love something life has brought you.
- At night, name three things you're grateful the day has ushered into your life.

*Gravity and wrinkles are fine with me.
They're a small price to pay for the new wisdom
inside my head and my heart.*

~Drew Barrymore

CHAPTER 2

Second Spring: Coping with the Shifts and Myths of Menopause

Honoring Hormones, Body Changes, and Intuitive Insights

One day at my monthly Radiant Wise Woman group, Karen confessed to the other women her struggles with the physical and emotional changes of perimenopause: "It's all so unpredictable. My period is super heavy for two days, but then it stops, followed by three months with no period at all. I feel extra emotional sometimes. Last week I asked my son and husband, 'How crazy do I seem to you?' I'm trying to keep it together, but I feel all out of whack."

Karen's story echoes that of many perimenopausal women. Others in the phase prior to menopause experience fewer changes, such as a skipped period a couple times one year, then a few normal cycles, then nothing. Still others are like Jackie, who said, "I turned fifty last August and thought I was prepared for changes. But last fall my period just stopped. I realize I'm not quite ready to be a woman in menopause. I still feel like I'm in my thirties, and sometimes I feel like I'm in my teens." Then, too, some women who have weathered perimenopause and menopause still have lingering issues years later, like brain fog or sleep difficulties.

Menopause is defined medically as a point in time when a woman has not menstruated for twelve months, although women commonly refer to menopause as the time between the onset of hormonal shifts and their last period. It is a significant transition in a woman's life, not only on a physical level but emotionally and spiritually as well. Because most women live with their menstrual cycles for thirty to forty years, letting go of the "fertile years" can feel as challenging as retiring or getting a divorce, evoking many of the same uncertainties. Whatever stage of the menopause passage you are in, you're probably facing many questions, such as: Who am I now? What's next? What am I grieving as I close this chapter of my life? However, despite its potential challenges, menopause is neither a pathology nor a disease process, although it can feel like one if you don't know how to support your body through this passage.

Most women experience menopause between ages forty and fifty-eight, the average age in the United States being fifty-one. Physical and emotional changes can begin years before the final menstrual period, in the transition phase called perimenopause, and may last for four to eight years.[1] The changes women encounter prior to and during menopause can be bewildering and challenging, with their hot flashes and anxiety often ignored or dismissed by medical professionals.

The experience of menopause varies widely from individual to individual. Some women sail through perimenopause and menopause without any issues, while others struggle with an onslaught of physical and mental changes. Weight gain, brain fog, mood swings, and lesser-known symptoms—migraines, joint aches, vaginal dryness, and digestive problems, as well as loss of sleep and energy—can continue into postmenopause, after periods end. Problems like depression can spike during perimenopause, especially among women predisposed to mood disorders. And many women endure hot flashes and night sweats, their own personal summer, as they wake up tangled in wet sheets or find their blouse drenched when they're about to make an important presentation. More Black, Latina, and Native American women report these vasomotor effects[2]; they can be hard to identify because women are not taught what a hot flash feels like, and consequently some think they're having panic attacks or heart problems, which can be frightening.

Many factors affect a woman's experience of menopause. Everything from family history to smoking and from frequency of exercise to stress levels in daily life can shape the impact of menopause. For instance, the Study of Women's Health Across the Nation (SWAN), which began in 1996, suggests that Black and Latina women begin perimenopause earlier; reach menopause at the median age of forty-nine, two years earlier than the national median age; experience more intense effects; and have a longer transition period than women of other ethnic backgrounds.[3]

How to Cope with the Transition of Menopause

During menopause, many women lose sleep, the ability to focus, and the energy needed to meet their responsibilities and accomplish their goals and dreams. They report that some days just taking a shower and getting dinner on the table is all they can handle. Here are some ways to cope with the changes that often accompany menopause.

Educate Yourself

If you have issues related to perimenopause, menopause, or hormonal imbalance that are problematic, learn all you can about available treatment options from a variety of trusted sources. Refer to the Resources section, beginning on page 167, for a list of recommended books and websites.

Monitor Your Health

Keep track of what's going on with your body, mind, and emotions, including menstrual patterns, hot flash patterns, and mood swings. Using a paper calendar or an app can make it easier to give your healthcare provider details that may otherwise be hard to remember. If you bring a thorough health history to an appointment and your practitioner brushes off your concerns, consider switching to one who specializes in perimenopause and menopause.

Practice Smart Self-Care

- Get enough exercise, eat a balanced diet, and consume alcohol only in moderation.
- Get sufficient sleep. Try to sleep at least seven hours each night without being interrupted by the 3:00 a.m. "hamster wheel of worry." A wide variety of online tools and apps use calming music, nature sounds, guided meditation, or brainwave binaural beats to help people relax, fall asleep, and stay asleep. Many women find that natural sleep aids—liquid magnesium, calming herbs like valerian and kava root, and essential oils such as lavender, ylang-ylang, or cedarwood—are effective.[4]
- Eat to support your adrenals, by eliminating sugar and processed foods and by consuming good fat (coconut oil, avocado, nuts) and colorful vegetables to stabilize glucose and insulin. Feed your helpful gut bacteria daily with nutrients such as cacao powder, flaxseed meal, blueberries, and naturally fermented foods.[5]

- Reduce stress as much as possible. If your stress is out of control, develop a simple mindfulness practice as an antidote to feeling overwhelmed. One enjoyable way to calm your nervous system and build immunity is by listening to nature sounds as you work or walk. Listening to a calming podcast such as *Meditative Story* can also shift your mind and body out of fight, flight, or freeze mode and into rest-and-restore mode.

Cultivate Community

Form a supportive group of women to talk to during this transition to help cope with the changes and feel less isolated. Reach out to others your age or older and ask them, "Is anybody else going through this?" Share solutions and resources, listen with compassion, and laugh together as much as possible to ease the journey.

Call on Your Inner Allies

Call on your inner allies, your three feminine archetypes—the Maiden, Queen, and Wise Woman—to guide you through menopause. Although Western society tells a pessimistic story about this transition (you're going to dry up, become a hag, never want sex again, and lose your value in society), they can help you tell a new story about life during and after menopause, revealing that women can be beautiful, active, and vibrant at any age—forty, fifty, sixty, seventy, eighty, and beyond.

For example, if you are a woman in perimenopause, likely in your forties—the Queen phase of life—and juggling a multitude of responsibilities, including nurturing many other people, you may find little time for self-care beyond an occasional manicure or massage. You may have become so accustomed to giving that you've forgotten how to receive. If you listen to your inner Queen, she will ask you whether you're trying to please others, putting yourself down, or overthinking. She may then remind you to stop these habits and replace them with self-nurturing behaviors such as asking for help from family and friends, finding a healthcare practitioner who respects and listens to you, and seeking support from other women.

Similarly, if during your postmenopausal years you feel stressed and sad about parts of your identity falling away, your inner Wise Woman can provide strength, offering this truth: we must be willing to let parts of our former self die in order to truly live. You may be searching for permission to do life your own way—to think what you think and say what you want. When you call on your Wise Woman to stand by your side, she will guide you through any confusion about your emerging identity and new goals until you can clearly voice your desires and take small steps, or even a big leap, onto a new path.

By calling on these feminine archetypes, your inner allies, you can transcend the limitations that others have set for you and access your courage, beauty, and strength to continue fulfilling your potential. And once you can redefine menopause and aging with their aid, you ease passage through the wisdom years not only for yourself but for women coming behind you.

The Hormone Question

The pharmaceutical industry has fostered a perception that women embrace hormone replacement as the answer to their menopause challenges. In the male-dominated medical community of the 1950s, gynecologist Robert A. Wilson referred to postmenopausal women as "castrates," elaborating on this theme in his 1966 best seller *Feminine Forever*. This

Second Spring

influential book, it later emerged, was backed by Wyeth, a pharmaceutical company eager to market hormone replacement therapy as the way to remain sexy after fifty. However, many women are wary of synthetic hormones, having been cautioned about the health risks of hormone replacement, including breast cancer.

Personally, I struggled with the decision about hormone replacement. When I was forty-eight, I remember waking up in the middle of the night to fling the covers off my sweat-drenched body. It felt as if some invisible force was slamming me from one wall to the other. Physically and emotionally exhausted, I pulled my journal from the bedside table and scribbled questions such as: What is wrong? How can I stop feeling so confused? Why can't I sleep?

The next morning in desperation I called a friend a few years older than me who suggested I might be going through the beginning stages of menopause. It was the late 1990s, and since the topic was still taboo, menopause was not discussed in major women's magazines. I scheduled an appointment with an internist, who listened to the description of my symptoms and quickly wrote me a prescription for Premarin, a synthetic estrogen replacement derived from horse urine. Since I was at a breaking point, I took the medication he recommended. It relieved my night sweats, but every morning when I opened the orange bottle of pills I felt queasy. At the time, I didn't recognize this reaction as a message from my intuition warning me that something was not right.

A year later I read about bio-identical hormone replacement therapy (HRT), which I assumed was a natural alternative to the synthetic hormones I was taking. I eagerly made an appointment with a local integrative medicine doctor, who recommended an estrogen patch, progesterone pills, and a testosterone cream. Three days after starting this routine I felt like myself again. Unaware of the growing body of research that discouraged prolonged use of this regimen, I stayed on it for fifteen years, often wondering, with increasing dread, if it was safe for me. I felt stuck. I didn't want to give up the benefits of a calmer mood and good sleep, but I was afraid of the negative long-term impact of HRT on my health as suggested by newly released findings. For example, Dr. Zach Bush, a renowned specialist in internal medicine and endocrinology, had found that women's bodies were not designed to interact with bio-identical hormones, and that putting growth hormones in stressed bodies could be a setup for cancer. He recommended hormone replacement therapy only as a short-term crutch to help women get through a challenging phase.[6]

Fortunately, while seeking help in navigating this dilemma, I met a medically trained professional who worked with women to establish a personalized approach to wellness based on Western medical science, Ayurvedic medicine, and homeopathy. With her guidance and a customized protocol, I was able to stop taking bio-identical hormones and clear my body of toxins.

I also modified my diet to accommodate the decrease in hormones, as Dr. Mindy Pelz, author of *The Menopause Reset*, advised women to do after age forty.[7] Sweets had been my go-to energy source for decades, but I gradually weaned myself off sugar to regulate my insulin levels. I strengthened my gut health and immune system with prebiotics and probiotics, and began eating a gluten-free and mostly plant-based diet. I had been avoiding carbohydrates, thinking that was a good way to maintain a healthy weight. But I learned that as we enter our forties and progesterone levels decline we need a balance of foods that supply progesterone, such as legumes, purple potatoes, hard squashes, root vegetables, citrus fruits, wild rice, and quinoa. By restricting carbohydrates, I had actually been depleting the progesterone I needed to help prevent hair loss, anxiety, and insomnia.[8] I also started taking capsules of maca, a plant cultivated in the Andes for at least three thousand years and found to be an effective remedy for female hormone imbalance, symptoms of menopause, weak bones, and depression.[9] In addition, I applied a progesterone cream derived from wild yams, and used a homeopathic remedy at bedtime to help me sleep soundly through the night.

It took eighteen months to rebuild my adrenals and develop a healthy equilibrium, but I became more resilient than ever. When I have a rare hot flash now, instead of seeing it as a problem I view it as a sign of the fire that stokes my inner passion. I remind myself that this is my feminine energy rising—*I'm a red hot mama*. I am committed to listening to my body and adapting my wellness protocol to maintain optimal health throughout the rest of my life.

We are all unique. My hope is that you will feel inspired to take charge of your wellness and trust you can find the answers that are right for you. Many opinions and recommendations can be found about hormone balance during menopause, but there is no one-size-fits-all approach. Ultimately, every woman must do what's right for her based on her body, beliefs, and lifestyle. If your current healthcare professional isn't supportive, don't hesitate to switch to someone better positioned to respond to your needs. It's okay to try a new approach or request a second opinion. Search for a specialist in menopause, a doctor or functional medicine practitioner who is experienced, compassionate, and willing to listen respectfully to your concerns, address your questions, find solutions that fit your needs, and help you get your life back.

Gifts of Menopause

In the United States alone, of the six thousand women who enter menopause every day, amounting to an estimated two million each year,[10] regrettably few appreciate or even recognize its gifts. In fact, for many this midlife transition is often met with dread and suffering. For others it is a time of confusion. This is due in part to the fact that women have learned to view menopause as merely a biological occurrence rather than a doorway to the Wise Woman years, a time of liberation and blossoming of a woman's deepest purpose.

Another reason women today are generally unaware of the gifts of menopause—despite Chinese medicine's references to it as a "second spring," the flowering of feminine potential and ripening of wisdom and creativity[11]—is because the experience has largely been misunderstood throughout the ages, based on fear of the Wise Woman and her power. This is evidenced by the persecution and slaughter of more than forty thousand female healers, midwives, and herbalists accused of witchcraft in Europe and Colonial America during the fifteenth through eighteenth centuries.[12] Since then, cultural shaming and silencing have continued to repress women, although this paradigm is now beginning to shift.

Second Spring

The truth is that menopause can indeed be a blessing. All the crazy things happening internally during menopause can serve as barometers encouraging us to listen to our bodies and teaching us about our desires and dreams. In fact, insights gleaned during menopause help some women resolve past traumas, leading to a new acceptance of themselves and their family relationships, as is evident from the following story disclosed by one of the women I interviewed.

This woman confided: "At the beginning of menopause, I fell head over heels in love with my best friend, a woman I'm now married to. Alongside this morphing of my social identity and self-image, I felt a profound surge toward choosing my own life path, my own creativity, and more. It wasn't an easy time. Everything ruled by hormones got scrambled. But when those hormones started to leave my system, I spiraled back to myself as a young woman, and my grief and rage showed me the places calling out to be healed—my desperately poor relationship to my body and acting out sexually with men. Wherever we need change, menopause will take us, and for me it presented a chance to heal what I couldn't face amidst the chaos of my life. I laugh a lot more now, and I really don't care what other people think of me."

The years beyond menopause hold the potential for another gift. While one of the prevailing myths of menopause claims that women's sex drive disappears at this time, the truth is that mature women can be newly awakened to passion, pleasantly surprised to discover their desire reaching new heights after menopause. This became evident to me when my friend Barbara and I were attending a business conference in California and went out for dinner one evening with a small circle of our close girlfriends. As often happened when we got together, the conversation turned to sexual pleasure. We huddled around the table long after the ice had melted in our drinks, riveted by Barbara's tales of erotic ecstasy, interrupted only by our squeals of laughter and cries to "tell us more!" Postmenopausal and inspired by her revelations, I began to explore my own potential for passion. (See chapter 7 for details of the multi-orgasmic life women can look forward to in their fifties, sixties, seventies, and beyond.)

The wisdom years can also bring an enhanced ability to see past outward appearances and be more intuitive and creative, as if a heavy curtain were pulled back, permitting you to look through a clear window. Christiane Northrup, MD, explains this phenomenon in her book *The Wisdom of Menopause*, where she indicates how, after menopause, two formerly female reproductive hormones—luteinizing hormone (LH) and follicular-stimulating hormone (FSH)— become neurotransmitters for the right (intuitive) side of the brain.[13] Following this conversion, women discover an increase in creativity, telepathic abilities, and visionary gifts that enrich their lives.

When I asked women to share their stories about perimenopause and menopause, one woman sent an email with this encouraging message: "I'm forty-eight years old and have been dealing with many of the physical symptoms of perimenopause for the last four or five years—hot flashes, mood swings that feel like hurricanes, and cramps. About a year ago I started going two or three months without a period, which brought on many new physical symptoms such as heartburn, sleeplessness, increased anxiety, and breast tenderness. I'm supporting myself through this life transition with weekly acupuncture, slowing down, prioritizing sleep, and daily movement outdoors. I'm eating more intuitively—no more dieting and the stress it causes. What has most helped me alter my perspective about this change and embrace the power of it is seeing perimenopause and menopause as a good thing. I finally like who I am becoming; it's a time in my life for me."

Due to their clearer perspective during the wisdom years, women can also experience enhanced self-confidence, increasingly trusting their own inner knowing instead of habitually yielding to authority figures. This is reflected in the actions of my client Lori when she faced a frightening medical situation. One crisp fall afternoon I was on the patio of a coffee shop sipping a creamy latte when Lori called, dissolving into tears as she told me, "I just left the gynecologist's office. She says I need a hysterectomy because I have fibroids, which might turn into cancer. But I don't have a good feeling about this doctor. She got irritated and cut me off when I asked questions." Lori had scheduled the appointment because, while in perimenopause, she'd begun having episodes of profuse vaginal bleeding. Now faced with this health predicament, she found that her self-reliance—a gift she had developed by calling on her Queen and Wise Woman energies—suddenly became crucial. Rather than defer to the doctor's opinion, as she might have done earlier in her life, Lori was determined to learn all she could about her available options.

Invigorated by this more empowered approach, she researched the pros and cons of various medical treatments for fibroids and sought a second opinion from a doctor she trusted. She eventually decided it was safe to monitor the situation without taking immediate action. Within two months, the bleeding had stopped and tests showed that the fibroids had shrunk significantly. Because she had followed her intuition, done due diligence, and made a carefully considered decision, she'd been able to avoid radical surgery. Lori was happy with this outcome but was even more pleased with herself for having taken responsibility for her own well-being, having embraced her Queen and listened to her Wise Woman self.

Perhaps one of the most powerful medicines we have—one that can keep us from getting sick, cure us, or harm us—is our belief system. What we tell ourselves can greatly impact our health. Examining our beliefs about menopause empowers us, when challenged, to explore solutions that ignite the joy of living in our bodies, confident that midlife and beyond can be the best years of our lives.

Honoring Sacred Exhaustion

During menopause and beyond, it is common to feel an exhaustion as challenging as any changes we've faced, yet it can shed light on a more fulfilling future. This dynamic became apparent to me following an encounter I had with a colleague and brilliant entrepreneur named Diane. While attending a statewide networking event in Birmingham, Alabama, I had the pleasure of hearing Diane deliver an inspiring keynote speech to several hundred women. After the event, we arrived at the elevator at the same time. She appeared poised, confident, and impeccably attired. "I loved your presentation today," I said. To my surprise, she burst into tears as she talked about her sleepless nights while juggling the demands of both a thriving business and two teenagers, often repeating the refrain "I'm just so tired."

As we spoke further, it became clear that she was living in fear of dropping one of the numerous balls in her life, and her critical inner voice was telling her she could not rely on anyone for help. Yet she wasn't willing to give up hope. We agreed to talk the following day, get to the root of her weariness, and assess its impact on her life.

To help Diane get an accurate picture of her commitments, I invited her to list her business activities and allocate each one to either the top, middle, or bottom of a pyramid to help prioritize their importance. We defined the three categories as follows:

Top: Cake

The activities you love doing

In Diane's case, it was writing,
speaking, and consulting with her clients.

Middle: Okay

*The activities you can do and may
be good at, but don't love doing*

For Diane, this was writing blog posts, compiling training manuals, buying gifts for employees, and leading weekly staff meetings.

Bottom: Cringe

The activities you hate doing

For Diane, this entailed making travel arrangements, conducting research for speaking engagements, and managing her client schedule.

The clarity that came from categorizing her work activities in this way prompted Diane to delegate her "cringe" and "okay" tasks to trusted employees who enjoyed doing them. She dedicated the time she had freed up to pursuits she had longed to do but could never fit into her schedule. She began writing her first book, engaging with new high-potential clients, accepting speaking gigs in fun locations, and planning escapes to the beach for rest and reflection. For the first time in her career, she could see her priorities clearly enough to envision how she wanted to spend the rest of her life and began setting positive intentions regarding her family, finances, fun, and serving as the visionary leader she was meant to be.

Many clients and women I have met while traveling have experienced similar chronic fatigue. I've come to view this condition as sacred exhaustion. Why sacred? Because when we're willing to listen to what it has to tell us we get a clearer view of ourselves and the horizon of our future.

Poet David Whyte tells an enlightening story about a time when he was bone tired in a way that affected every part of his life. He had been working with a nonprofit organization, and after an embarrassing incident at work one day—due to a lapse of memory stemming from his exhaustion—he went home and called on the wise counsel of a dear friend, the renowned Benedictine monk Brother David Steindl-Rast. With the two seated at Whyte's kitchen table, Whyte asked his spiritual brother to speak to him of exhaustion, desperately wanting to know what was at the root of it.

The kind monk said, "You know, David, the antidote to exhaustion is not necessarily rest. The antidote to exhaustion is wholeheartedness."

If you're often exhausted and feel your health and well-being are being compromised, you can arrive at the needed remedy by exploring the following questions: Are you living your life with your whole heart engaged, or are you just going through the motions of being alive? Are you emotionally available, or do you feel guarded and emotionally numb? Are you saying yes to things you would rather say no to? Are you working at a job you don't love? Are you longing to put some of your skills and talents to use in new ways? What desires are you aching to express? What dreams are you longing to fulfill? If you're willing to ask yourself what it is you want and respond to promptings from your heart, you will see your energy respond in kind.

In her audiobook *The Late Bloomer,* Dr. Clarissa Pinkola Estés also describes the tiredness we feel that is not remedied by rest, a fatigue that comes from the inability to move forward with actions that can bring new life.[14] Estés relates the story of an old woman who is told she shouldn't hike to a nearby stream because it's too scary and dangerous. In response, with initiative and determination she makes herself a pair of red boots that end up providing the sturdiness she needs to climb toward the stream, where she fills her bucket with water. When we are stuck in utter tiredness, we can feel lethargic and lost, torn between listening to our inner taskmaster and succumbing to weariness. But when we pause to discern the stronger call of what our hearts are longing for, we can find the sweet spot between surrendering to life as it unfolds and full-on engagement. Then, as we pull on our version of the red boots and step forward, we begin to feel recharged by an energized sense of wonder and curiosity.

BREATHING SPACE

My body is a miracle.

When I listen to my body, it shows me what it needs.

My intuition is getting clearer day by day.

I can discern when to pull on my red boots,
walk to the river, and fill my bucket.

Second Spring

PRACTICE

Assess Your Beliefs about Aging

To better understand your beliefs about menopause and aging, ask yourself the following questions. Then consider how your answers may be impacting your views on menopause and aging.

How do I think my aging body will affect my life?

Do I believe that getting older is like having a disease?

Do I assume that getting older means I can no longer be vibrant and sexy?

Am I afraid of my body and its changes?

Do I expect to be challenged by disease or physical limitation as I age?

Do I think that only doctors have the ability to heal me?

What do I believe about my ability to heal?

In regard to my health and well-being, how might I be giving away my power?

PRACTICE

Energy Vampires Quiz—What Is Draining You?

One of the quickest ways to amplify your energy and radiance is by taking an inventory of your life to identify what gives you energy and what zaps your energy. Your responses to this quiz will reveal aspects of your life that are draining you and how best to nurture, protect, and increase your energy.

Read the statements below and give yourself a "1" for each statement that rings true for you. Then add up your final score and, based on the concluding segment of this practice, see what that tells you.

Relationships

____ There are people in my life who consistently drain my energy.

____ I have unreturned phone calls, emails, or letters that need to be addressed.

____ I lack quality friendships in my life.

____ I want a romantic partner.

____ There is a relationship in my life that I need to end.

____ I want a better relationship with my child (or another family member).

____ There is a conversation I dread having, and it causes me stress and anxiety.

____ There is someone in my life who consistently irritates, frustrates, or annoys me.

____ I long to be part of a loving and supportive community.

Environment

____ My home is cluttered and disorganized.

____ My car needs to be cleaned or repaired.

____ My wardrobe needs updating, alteration, or cleaning.

____ I'd like to live in a different geographic location.

___ I have appliances that need repair or upgrading.
___ I need to decorate my home in a more nurturing way.
___ I need to create a quiet place for doing my work.

Body, Mind, and Spirit
___ I eat food that isn't good for me.
___ It's been too long since I've been to the dentist.
___ I don't get the sleep I need to feel fully rested.
___ I'd like to exercise regularly but never seem to find the time.
___ I have a health concern for which I've avoided getting help.
___ There are books I'd love to read but haven't found the time for.
___ My thoughts often sabotage me.
___ I lack a spiritual or religious practice in my life.

Work
___ My work is stressful and leaves me exhausted at the end of the day.
___ My office is so disorganized and messy that I have trouble finding what I need.
___ I'm avoiding confronting a problem at work.
___ I'm working too hard for too little money.
___ I'm not as computer literate as I need to be, and it hinders my productivity.

____ I need to delegate specific tasks, but I'm unable to let go of control.

____ With email, voicemail, snail mail, and texts, I'm on information overload.

____ I spend too many hours at work but never feel like it's finished.

Money

____ I pay my bills late.

____ I charge less for my services than I'm worth.

____ I don't have a plan for my financial future.

____ My credit rating is not what I'd like it to be.

____ I don't have a regular savings plan.

____ I don't have adequate insurance coverage.

____ I have debts that need to be paid off.

____ **Final Score**

What Your Score Tells You

Score 0–12: Congratulations! You're running on clean energy most of the time.
You've eliminated many energy vampires from your life. You wake up feeling pretty good most days. You get a lot of the important things done and still have time for fun, but some days you feel overwhelmed. You want to feel amazing every day, but you're not sure how to create reserves of time and energy to tap in to.

Score 13–25: *Your engine is misfiring, and your tank is getting low.*
You're starting to drop some balls. You feel weighed down by guilt about family and work. It seems like you have to do everything without help, and you resent it. You wake up at night worried about your to-do list. You feel out of control, as if your life is running you.

Score 26–39: *You're in the express lane speeding toward Burnout City.*
You're constantly on edge. Little things feel overwhelming. You worry every day that you've forgotten something important or that you're letting things fall through the cracks. People often comment that you look tired. You know you need to pay attention to your body's warnings to slow down, but you are too overwhelmed with commitments.

If your score is 16 or higher, it's time to start eliminating the energy zappers you've been tolerating, so that you can regain your energy. You don't have to tackle everything right away. Small, deliberate steps in the direction of your desires will provide momentum and inspire you to keep going. Remember, no matter how high your score is, there's a way to get off the psycho path and onto the scenic path.

*I used to have a handle on life,
but it broke off when menopause started.*

~Anonymous

CHAPTER 3

Honey, Read This: For the Men

Sharing Concerns about Menopause

Men typically don't think it's necessary to know about menopause until the women they love need their understanding and support because they have started experiencing the confusing midlife changes that can derail their lives. Then, living with them in the throes of menopause, men often wonder how to survive this physical and emotional roller coaster with their relationships intact. Thus, learning early on about menopause can be a smart investment in a man's future happiness.

In her song "PMS Blues," Dolly Parton aptly expresses the challenges of being, and being around, a woman in a hormonal storm:

> I don't even like myself, but it's something I can't help
> I got those god almighty, slap somebody pms blues
> Most times I'm easy going, some say I'm good as gold
> But when I'm pms I tell ya, I turn mean and cold
>
> Those not afflicted with it are affected just the same
> You poor old men didn't have to grin and say
>   "I feel your pain"...
> You know you must forgive us for we care not what we do
> I got those can't stop crying, dishes flying pms blues

But you know we can't help it
We don't even know the cause
But as soon as this part's over, then comes the menopause
Oh, lord, oh, lord

We're going to always be a heap of fun
Like the devil taking over my body, suffering,
    suffering, suffering
Everybody's suffering, huh?[1]

Men who try to help women entering menopause are often puzzled because they don't understand what's happening or are frustrated because their best efforts have little or no positive impact. They may wonder what's wrong with their partner or their eyes may glaze over when she describes in great detail her latest spat with a relative or friend. While most men have no idea how women's hormones influence their physical and emotional health, many women themselves don't know much about menopause until it affects them. Even its precursor, perimenopause, often takes women by surprise. Typically it starts in their forties, but actor Gillian Anderson, famous for playing Margaret Thatcher in *The Crown*, went through perimenopause in her early thirties, experiencing severe disorientation.[2] So it's no wonder both men and women can become confused during this time.

Many women view the menopausal years as an exasperating experience they have to suffer alone. They often think they must pretend they are fine. And even if they want to talk about it with their partners they don't know how, especially if their symptoms are not outwardly visible and they fear their partners, considering their complaints unjustified, will be dismissive.

Men, for their part, often have an urge to fix things for their partners in this situation, hoping conditions will get back to normal. But in order to be truly helpful they may need more information about how menopause affects women and the most effective kinds of support to offer. The following insights and suggestions will help.

What It Is Like to Be Her

If you are a man reading this, to better communicate with your partner it might be helpful to take a closer, more intimate look at what women in this major life transition think and feel. Here are some of the thoughts and feelings women shared with me about their experiences with menopause:

> "These are rough times. We are aging and seeing the effects of that on our bodies—wrinkles, gray hairs, sagging, unexplained weight gain, and a lack of energy. Then come the hormonal changes. It all feels confusing, awful, and scary. Menopause is like the teen years, except one hundred times worse."

> "Literally, one moment you're fine and then the next you feel like you're in a vat of boiling water, as if the rug has been pulled out from underneath you."

> "When I was in my early thirties, I was confident—the mother of a toddler, in a strong marriage, with the best job I'd ever had, doing lots of exercise, and full of energy. Today, I'm fifty and have lost all my self-confidence, my libido, and my energy and optimism. I'm confused, frustrated, and scared about the future."

"For me, the hardest part is the crushing anxiety and the acid reflux, plus being permanently tired but pretending I'm okay."

"I feel like the police chief in *Jaws*. When I realized what was happening, I wanted to tell my boyfriend to go find me a bigger boat. There is so much going on in my brain and my body, I can't quite grasp it all. Mostly there is the feeling that I'm not myself anymore, which can be hard to articulate."

"I could scream and pig out on chocolate and run and cry because it seems all the responsibility is mine and I should just relax. I can't freakin' relax when there's so much to do and it feels like I'm the only one doing anything."

"Don't pressure me for sex while I'm going through this. I still want to have sex but not under pressure."

"I'm going through a life-changing experience in my physical body that affects my emotional health and my self-esteem. I already feel bad about myself. Don't make it worse by making negative comments about how I look."

What You Can Do

Men enjoy winning, but women often don't tell them how to win in the game of living with menopause, which can be frustrating for everyone involved. Winning in such instances can depend on your partner telling you what she needs; you responding by doing things that are helpful; and your partner telling you how much she appreciates your assistance. It requires communicating with each other and cooperating to get through this difficult time together.

I asked women to share their game rules by responding to the question: What can a man do to help when you're on the menopause roller coaster? Based on their responses, some strategies for winning are the following:

- Give her time alone for quiet self-reflection, perhaps even by running the bathwater and putting a candle and bath salts by the tub.
- Comment on admirable things you notice about her or fond memories you have about your times together.
- Do chores around the house more frequently to help lower her stress.
- Rub her feet after work to help her relax and feel cared for.
- Be romantic. Play a song the two of you love, and ask her to dance. Or take her out to dinner and ask about her dreams or aspirations.
- Research beneficial treatments, such as acupuncture. Discuss them and, if she's interested, offer to make appointments for her with practitioners.
- Let her know you find her attractive and are interested in having sex, without pressuring her to engage in it.
- Provide space for her. Periodically put down your phone, toolbox, or TV remote and listen to her. Ask if there is anything you can do for her, and offer to do what she requests.

Your Cheat Sheet

Here are five things to remember to do so you won't make matters worse:

1. *Stop* hiding out or ignoring her.
   Start admitting you're frustrated.
2. *Stop* waiting for her to explain it all to you.
   Start learning about it yourself.
3. *Stop* thinking her symptoms are her fault.
   Start researching and offering information on beneficial treatments.
4. *Stop* criticizing her actions (such as complaining about her blasting the A/C).
   Start encouraging her and doing small things to help (like keeping a sweater nearby).
5. *Stop* trying to fix her (through instructing or "mansplaining").
   Start asking what she needs (such as time alone or help with dishes, laundry, or the children).

The women I surveyed about their menopausal years often expressed gratitude for the patience and kindness shown by the men in their lives. For example, one woman said, with tears in her eyes, "I'd be completely lost without him. It's actually quite scary how much I rely on his support." Another woman told me, "My husband is great. He puts up with my moods; he understands why on some days I'm in pain or grumpy. He cooks, helps clean, and makes me laugh a lot." Communication and consideration together help partners better weather menopause.

Honey, Read This

How to Handle Complaints

Anytime your partner is in distress and you feel frustrated or trapped when she complains, try this tactic: listen to her, make a supportive statement, and then ask how she plans to handle the troublesome issue in the future, ultimately letting her know that you are there for her. Here are some examples.

- When she complains about hot flashes or lack of sleep, you could say, "I'm sorry you feel bad. That sounds hard to deal with. What do you think is going on?"

- When she complains after a depressing visit with her doctor, you could say, "He said that, really? It must have been difficult to hear. What are you going to do? Whatever it is, I'll support you."

- When she complains about an upsetting encounter with a family member, you could say, "I can see why you're upset. I'm on your side. Any idea how you'll deal with this if it happens again?"

Once you have assured your partner of your support for her plan to move forward, ask if she would like you to get involved or just listen. Although it's hard to resist the impulse to grab the reins while watching someone you love make choices you wouldn't make, a carefully posed question, asked with genuine concern, can help her see ways to maintain control of her destiny while still feeling supported. Think of it this way: you're turning on a light so she can see how to get out of a dark room.

What's the Payoff?

Although menopause can be a difficult time for women and their partners, the good news is that after menopause most women feel more vibrant, confident, and energetic, as well as less worried because they are better able to solve problems of all kinds, from minor daily dilemmas to big challenges. Changes of this nature can be enormously beneficial to relationships going forward.

The payoff for your willingness to understand more about menopause and help your partner through this transition is that you get to be a hero—to bring your problem-solving skills, strength, steadiness, and caring to a perplexing and troublesome situation. Your support will be a priceless gift, and your partner will have new appreciation for you. You might even overhear her bragging to her girlfriends about what a great guy you are. Your heroism, combined with her deepened respect and affection for you, is sure to strengthen and enhance your relationship.

BREATHING SPACE

My partner and I are on the same team.

When she feels better, I feel better.

Honey, Read This

PRACTICE

Can You Hear Me?

You cannot always resolve your partner's issues with menopause, but you can provide physical and emotional support. The most important thing you can do is ensure that communication does not break down. Understanding each other's way of talking and listening is a giant step toward keeping lines of communication open.

Women frequently complain that men don't listen to them. But often when women say, "You aren't listening," and men counter with, "Yes, I am," the men are right. What causes this misunderstanding, and what can you do to fix it? Deborah Tannen, communications expert and author of the best-selling book *You Just Don't Understand,* identifies the roots of this predicament as differing conversational styles and points to two clues: body talk and "listener-noise."[3]

Body talk differences, Tannen explains, are a major obstacle. When listening to others, girls and women tend to face them directly, eyes anchored on their faces. Boys and men more often sit at angles to others and look around the room, periodically glancing at them, showing they are attuned to the conversation by mirroring their movements. Men's tendency to face away from others while listening can give women the impression they aren't listening when, in fact, they are.

Listener-noise contrasts, in Tanner's view, can be just as misleading. To show they are listening, women make noises, such as "Mmm," "Uh-huh," and "Yeah," while men more often give silent attention. Women who expect a stream of listener noise interpret silent attention as no attention at all and can become frustrated at what they see as lack of communication with a partner. For example, whenever one woman told her husband she wanted to talk to him he would lie on the floor, close his eyes, and wrap his arm over his face. This signaled to her that he was taking a nap. But he claimed he was listening extra hard, insisting that lying down and covering his eyes actually helped him concentrate on what she was saying. He felt attacked by her accusations and believed that to change his behavior would be to admit fault. Ultimately the woman learned about the differences in women's and men's habitual ways of positioning themselves in conversation and explained them to her husband. The next time she told him she wanted to talk, he lay down on the floor and covered his eyes. When she felt unheard, her familiar negative reaction, she reassured herself that he really was listening. Then he sat up and looked at her. Thrilled, she asked why. He said, "You like me to look at you when we talk, so I'm trying to do it." Having come to see their differences as habits rather than right and wrong conduct, he had chosen to alter his behavior.

Another source of misunderstanding communication styles lies in the fact that female and male brains are wired differently. The female brain has more wiring in areas that play a role in social cognition and verbal communication. That may be why women are typically better at empathizing with others and tend to use more expressive language. The male brain has less wiring between verbal centers and those of their emotions and memories, which may contribute to men having less interest in conversations.[4]

Women and men also have different expectations about communication. For women, talk creates intimacy, making them feel vulnerable while revealing their emotions and thoughts—and pushed away if they are ignored. But for men talk signifies independence and status; being perceived as a listener can therefore make a man feel controlled or put down, like a child listening to an adult or an employee to a boss. It is no wonder that bonds between men are based less on talk and more on doing things together. Since they don't view talk as the cement that binds a relationship, men don't know what kind of talk women want, and they don't miss it when it isn't there.

Understanding that male-female communication issues are largely prompted by gender differences rather than personal agendas makes it easier to learn new behaviors. Even five or ten minutes of listening can profoundly enhance your relationship with your partner, as well as your mutual emotional and physical well-being. To support your partner throughout menopause so both of you are happier, incorporate the following practice into your day at least several times a week.

1. Put aside whatever you're doing, and sit down with your partner.
2. Set a timer for 5–10 minutes.
3. Listen to her without interrupting.
4. Nod your head and make listening sounds ("Uh-huh," "Hmm") when appropriate.
5. If she stops talking, say, "Tell me more" or "What else?"
6. When the timer dings, say, "Thank you" then lean in with at least brief eye contact.

*If you want to see the brave,
look at those who can forgive.*

~Bhagavad Gita

CHAPTER 4

Flying Free on Wings of Forgiveness
Releasing Destructive Patterns and Old Hurts

Authentic forgiveness is challenging, and staying open can be a divinely inspired act of courage. These insights were revealed during a retreat I led in Costa Rica with women from around the world who had come for a week of rest, play, and transformation. On the day they arrived, they braided fresh tropical flowers into their hair and adorned themselves with colorful sarongs and scarves, each channeling her inner Maiden and having fun getting to know the others. The next morning we began the day by forming a circle on comfy wicker couches in the outdoor living space. We felt the cool stone floor on our bare feet; a gentle breeze kissed our faces; and we feasted our eyes on the gorgeous sunrise with pink rays of light breaking through wispy clouds. From across the valley, the indigo boulders of Mount Chirripó, sacred to the Maya, watched over us with their quiet strength.

We started with a sound healing—clear tones ringing from a crystal bowl—to help soften our hearts. Next each woman spoke about what had opened up for her since arriving at the retreat. For one woman, it was the joy of waking up to see a parade of peacocks by the pool. Another woman shared her sense of wonder about a dream she'd had the night before of flying like an eagle. Yet another said she felt she had finally found the sisters she'd always longed for. As each spoke, the others listened with empathy and acceptance. We then turned our attention to letting go of our emotional ties with the past.

The Wise Woman years present a golden opportunity to free ourselves of the baggage we have carried and, through forgiveness, release destructive family patterns that may go back generations, so we don't have to replay traumas that have scarred and shamed us. Because it's our natural state to know ourselves as innocent, unburdened by guilt and regret, both our Maiden and our Wise Woman selves rush in to help as soon as we make the choice to heal. The Wise Woman offers her gifts of discernment and resolve to assist us in completing our unfinished business. With the heaviness lifted, our Maiden dances in, bringing us a sense of delight and freedom.

We may first approach forgiveness rationally, with thoughts like: "I'm going to forgive because I should. It's the right thing to do. I know I need to forgive. I already forgave him so there's no need to revisit that." But thinking on its own doesn't set the heart free. We also have to feel our way to forgiveness and freedom. To move in this direction, throughout the retreat we worked with the four primary elements of nature—fire, earth, air, and water. On the first day, we focused on fire, which represents both the healing power of the sun and the inner passion that illuminates our path. The intensity of our internal fire can help us burn through unresolved life experiences, release the past, and align with our higher mission in life.

So I invited each woman to write down her past troubling experiences and reflect on ways they might be weighing her down. As the women wrote about the experiences they wanted to release, I pulled out my journal and prepared to explore a pain stored in my heart. I closed my eyes, took a few deep breaths, and within minutes I was a six-year-old again, revisiting a life-changing moment when my father came home from work and announced that he had a new game to play. He put me on top of the tall white Frigidaire in our kitchen, stood facing me, and said, "Jump, and I'll catch you!" The distance between us was probably no more than four feet, but to me it was a gaping chasm. I pulled my knees up under my chin and wrapped my arms around my skinny legs, trembling but thinking that if I made myself smaller maybe I wouldn't crash onto the kitchen floor. I looked to my right and saw my mother intently chopping onions on the red Formica counter, not looking at me or saying a word. I let my legs dangle over the refrigerator door, squeezed my eyes shut, and imagined myself safely in my father's arms. As I leaned forward and opened my eyes, ready to jump, what I saw broke my heart. My father had folded his arms and taken a step backward. Decades later in therapy, I realized the "jumping game" had taught me to believe that life isn't safe and that men can't be trusted. And at the retreat I dug deeper into this memory to pull out the roots of the pain related to my father, who had been missing in action for most of my life because of his destructive behavior around alcohol, women, and gambling.

After dinner that first day of the retreat, we held a fire ceremony of forgiveness to release the experiences we had written about. As we stood around the glowing fire pit, each of us, including myself, read our list of unresolved life experiences then tossed the paper into the flames, feeling both relief from the burdens we had been carrying and the compassion that was helping us view these old hurts with new eyes.

Turning Off the Pain Switch

All of us have stories of difficulties and disappointments, often in our closest relationships, and we inadvertently keep the pain alive when we feed these stories with our attention. Feelings of cynicism or anger about past situations signal parts of our lives calling out for forgiveness. When left unresolved, such feelings can become toxic to our systems. In fact, bitterness, the most potent poison generated in the body, is often at the root of physical pain.

Neuroscience studies show that physical pain is a short-lived neurological experience, but re-created over and over it becomes chronic. One factor that triggers such pain, turning the "pain switch" on, is the interaction between stress hormones, neurotransmitters, and our emotions.[1] People struggling with chronic physical pain can find this switch by locating the origin of the pain—through remembering when they first experienced it—and by identifying the emotion that may have triggered it, such as fear, shame, or anger.

For example, I suffered from migraine headaches every month for over forty years. Searching for relief, I recalled the first time I had felt piercing pain behind my right eye. My periods had just started; my parents' marriage was strained because of financial worries; and I knew that my father was having extramarital affairs. After drinking heavily one night, he made an inappropriate sexual advance toward me while my mother was in the kitchen. I pushed his hand away and looked up to see my mother standing silently in the doorway. Overcome with shame, I experienced my first migraine a few days later. In therapy sessions as an adult, I discovered that my pain was being activated by the shame I carried from that embarrassing experience as a twelve-year-old girl. To break the cycle of debilitating pain by turning off the pain switch, I realized that I needed not only to forgive my father but also to honor my innocence and forgive myself.

If you're suffering from chronic physical pain, you may find it fruitful to explore the possibility of an emotional trigger. Should you find one, consider whether forgiveness, of yourself or someone else or both of you, will help turn off the pain switch.

Forgiveness for Healing

You no longer need to be defined by past events that don't support your happiness if you engage your Wise Woman self as an ally in releasing them through forgiveness. When doing this, remember that forgiveness is neither about being good nor something you do for others. Rather, the purpose of forgiveness is to heal yourself so you can move on.

A good way to start this process is by better understanding the reasons for and effects of past painful events. If something traumatic happened to you when you were young, most likely no one explained its cause or its effects on you. Past trauma may still make little sense to you, especially if you've continued to look at it through the same lens as when you were younger. However, with the aid of your Wise Woman self you can now gain a new perspective from a more inclusive level of awareness. For instance, if you were mistreated as a child, invite your Wise Woman self to show you the truths behind the resulting trauma by asking her questions such as: What life lesson was this experience supposed to deliver to me? Why, from a higher dimensional perspective, did it happen? Asking such questions can lead to profound insights, permitting you to see why certain people have been a part of your life or how particular experiences taught you about self-reliance, overcoming shame, or acceptance.

When you connect with your Wise Woman self, she will offer you the power to compose new stories about past traumatic events as a means of personal liberation. For instance, consider the old story you're telling yourself about a disturbing experience. (It was my fault. There's something wrong with me. I can't trust anyone.) Now notice how that old story impacts you. (Such beliefs are limiting. They close my heart. They deplete my energy.) Then become aware of the new, truer story your Wise Woman whispers. (There is nothing wrong with me. I am safe now. I have allies to help me face this.) Creating new stories about past traumas in alliance with your Wise Woman allows you to see yourself as a heroine who overcomes obstacles and chooses to move toward a brighter future.

Ancestors as Allies

Ancestors can also be powerful allies in seeking forgiveness. Recently I took steps in my quest to fully forgive my father when a friend introduced me to Vassa, a wise, intuitive healer who taught me that connecting to our ancestors can be useful. A few minutes into our first conversation, she said, "Your ancestors struggled, fought, and made love to get you here. When you connect to their energy field, information will come through to help you on your life journey." She recommended a thirteen-minute ritual for me to engage in every day during the first week of each month.

Initially, I wasn't sure about doing this. After all, it had been my goal as an adult to escape the destructive patterns

Flying Free on Wings of Forgiveness

my ancestors had passed down. But with Vassa claiming that I could benefit from listening to them, I decided to try the ritual as an experiment. I gathered what I needed for it: five small cups, a pitcher of water, votive candles, and a clock. Then for seven consecutive nights I sat in front of a small table on which I had placed framed photos of my grandparents, mother, older sister, and father, with one cup and one votive candle in front of each. I began by closing my eyes for a moment and then opening them to gaze at the photo of each ancestor who had died. Vassa had instructed me to thank them for the gifts they had given me and ask them for any help I needed in my life. I first thanked Memaw, my father's mother, for always creating a warm, inviting home and feeding us from her big garden. I moved down the line, thanking each relative until I got to the photo of my father, fresh-faced and smiling in his marine uniform. As in life, he was the hardest for me to connect with. I noticed myself leaning back in the chair to put more distance between us. With my heart pounding, I poured water from the pitcher into his cup for refreshment and lit the candle to bring in light and energy. In a shaky voice, I offered a few words of love and thanks, but I was just going through the motions; inside, I felt nauseated. Doubts and questions flooded my mind: He had never shown up for me. He had been selfish and self-centered. *What help could he possibly have for me now?* At the same time, I knew the churning in my stomach came from the anger I had pushed down for decades and that now was the time to deal with it. I grabbed an old tennis racket and, with tears burning my eyes, hit the bed with it, feeling the thwack reverberate through my body and hearing jolting questions loosen from deep inside: Where were you when I needed you? Why were you so mean to me?

The second night I found it a little easier to connect internally with my father. This time I asked if he wanted me to give him anything special. I heard "A deck of cards" in my mind and recalled how he had loved to play hearts and poker. He also asked me to get him a cigarette and glass of whiskey. This was definitely a test since I had hated his drinking and smoking habits, and certainly didn't want to encourage them now. He had started smoking in third grade and was a chain smoker all his life, eventually dying of lung cancer. And his drinking had led to abusiveness in our home. But a little voice inside said, *Why not just give him what he asked for?* I rummaged through a kitchen cupboard, found a cigarette I had saved in case of a beesting and an old unopened bottle of Maker's Mark Bourbon. I poured him a shot, put the cards and cigarette on the table in front of his picture, and went to bed.

The next morning I woke to the sweet, earthy fragrance of roasting peanuts, although I had no idea where it was coming from. The aroma stayed with me all morning, wafting through the air at odd times while I did yoga poses, ate breakfast, and fed my cat. Finally, curiosity moved me to send Vassa an email asking: "Can you tell me what's up with the roasted peanuts?"

She replied that the smell of smoke or roasted food was a sign that one's ancestors are near. So I asked them, "Okay, do you have something to tell me?" The message that came through was an inner knowing that my father had the soul of an artist. I sensed that he had been sensitive as a boy. His father had gotten drunk every night, and he had been mercilessly bullied by his older brothers, who had been jealous of him for being their mother's favorite. I now felt his wounding—how afraid he had been of his brothers, how sad he had been about his father, and how his shame and confusion had affected him. I felt moved to pull out an unopened box my mother had given me after his death. Under layers of tissue paper, I discovered his art supplies—an assortment of fine brushes, paper, and dried tubes of paint. Chills went up my back as I moved my hand across the brushes and thanked him for his artistic talent.

On the sixth night, it was much easier to connect with my father. I said to him, "I love you," and felt a sweetness between us. I realized I had been a little girl the last time I said those words to him and meant them.

Since that day I've felt lighter and happier. I can remember the difficult moments with my father, but they no longer have a negative charge. My Wise Woman self has helped me see our relationship from a higher perspective. I'm clear now that we agreed, on a soul level, to play out specific roles in this lifetime. Even though he was too wounded to give me what I needed as a child, I see that my experiences with him helped me learn about compassion, boundaries, and claiming my power as a woman. By doing this work, I learned that I have the choice to stop the old cycle of blame and separation and that once I do, pain will dissolve into the gifts of deeper insight and compassion.

Self-Forgiveness for Ultimate Freedom

Self-forgiveness goes hand in hand with the desire to be fully free, a connection able to be seen and valued in our wisdom years. The honoring of this connection provided a particularly poignant experience at our retreat in Costa Rica. After we all had offered forgiveness to others during our releasing ceremony, we gathered by the fire, our hands warmed by cups of lemongrass mint tea, to share our thoughts. As if delivering a confession, Delia said, in a quivering voice, "I feel like I forgave a lot of people in my life. I forgave my father for taking his life when I was eleven. I forgave my brother for abusing me. But the one person I can't seem to forgive is myself." Every woman there nodded with understanding, relating to the pattern of self-blame.

Sensing a shared desire to release this core wound, I led the group through a simple yet potent self-forgiveness practice, which turned out to be one of the most transformative experiences they had that week. (See "Essential Steps to Self-Forgiveness" on page 79.)

When you can say with sincerity, "Thank you for what I have experienced; I forgive everyone, including myself; I claim all the gifts that have emerged from the darkness" and really feel it, you will know the ultimate freedom of being unhooked from the behavior and actions of others. To achieve this, it is worth taking risks—the risk of going on a soul retrieval expedition for the wounded part of you, the risk of speaking up for your innocent self, the risk of releasing hurt from your identity. Your reward is taking back your real life, bringing it to light, and living it fully as you become a vital expression of the woman you were born to be.

BREATHING SPACE

I help my inner child feel safe with me.

Everything that has happened is promoting my growth into the person I came here to be.

I choose to set my heart free by forgiving.

PRACTICE

Essential Steps to Forgiving Others

1. Picture the person you want to forgive standing in front of you. See the person as a child, innocent and hoping for love.

2. Remind yourself that you're both precious beings who agreed to create a life lesson together. Trust that you chose this lesson for the highest good of both of you.

3. Send a beam of love to the person's heart. Imagine a pink light entering their heart. Visualizing this for even a few seconds is effective.

4. See this person through eyes of pure love, or with the eyes of God/Spirit.

5. Imagine your own heart expanding and filling with golden light, even if just for a few seconds.

6. Say the words: "I forgive you. I release you. I let you go." Repeat this vow as many times as necessary until you feel at peace.

7. See yourself tearing up the life contract you had with this person. Then imagine yourself burning or burying the pieces.

PRACTICE

Essential Steps to Self-Forgiveness

1. Picture your younger self standing in front of you as a little girl, innocent and hoping for love.
2. Remind yourself that you're a precious being who now has an opportunity to learn an important life lesson. Trust that learning this lesson is for your highest good and that of everyone else involved.
3. Send a beam of love to your young self, imagining a pink light entering her heart. Visualizing this for even a few seconds is effective.
4. See her through eyes of pure love, or with the eyes of God/Spirit.
5. Imagine your younger self reaching out her hand to you and you taking it in yours.
6. Ask her, "What do you want me to know?" Listen closely to her answers.
7. Respond to her, repeating anything she asks you to say.
8. Tell her, "I love you. It wasn't your fault." Repeat this message as many times as is necessary until you feel at peace.

*Our wounds are often the openings
into the best and most beautiful part of us.*

~David Richo

CHAPTER 5

Chaos to Calm

Letting Your Wounds Become Your Wisdom

Times of turmoil test our inner strength, but they can also be times of great growth and transformation. I recall how one winter day in my twenties I was canoeing down a river with a friend when we hit a huge boulder buried under churning rapids and were thrown from the boat. An icy gasp caught in my throat as the leaden water darkened over me. The sharp granite tore at my fingers and arms as I fought to pull myself up the rock's jagged face. The harder I exerted myself, the more trapped I became in a swirling vortex forcing me deeper under the surface with each passing second. I had no idea how long I had been underwater, but my lungs were screaming for air. As the last molecules of oxygen burned up, I felt a sudden involuntary lurch of fear. But then, like a steel spring uncoiling, the whirlpool catapulted me out of its deadly trap. I gulped in the sharp, sweet air and thrashed my way to the riverbank, exhausted yet relieved. Similarly, sometimes it feels as if *life* is crashing over us and we can't catch our breath. An accident, divorce, bankruptcy, betrayal, or dire diagnosis, for instance, can threaten to drown us. We get messages from everywhere telling us to avoid the pain of traumatic experiences and instead buy, exercise, work, or eat our way through them. But the avoidance strategies we adopt for coping tend to prolong the pain, which ultimately keeps us in turmoil, unable to reach the serenity of resolution.

We are meant to deal with the chaos of existence. The moment we're born, our life force, like a river coursing toward the ocean, moves us from the chaos ever closer to our true home—the calm achieved through greater awareness and appreciation of the gifts of life. An apt image of this state was described to me by a friend who believes her horse, Dreamer, often answers her questions. When I told my friend I was writing a book for women forty and better, she volunteered to ask Dreamer: "Do you have a message for the readers of this book?" She received the following words from Dreamer: "When horses drink from a river, we never ask where we are in that river, if we are at the beginning or middle or end. We drink. We splash the current on our hooves. We are grateful for the stream that gives to us. Hold your heart like a beautiful crystal, precious beyond measure. You are timeless." This experience of radiance unbound by notions of time or place is accessible to us when we have attended to our pain and life lessons. Ignoring these, we cannot achieve the growth necessary to let our wounds become our wisdom.

Dark Night of the Soul

Ten years after my near-drowning experience I faced an even darker time because of a wrenching divorce and nasty custody battle. The same panic I had felt in the freezing river became a chronic companion as I struggled to navigate this unknown territory. During the divorce and legal battles, I felt utterly alone dealing with the situations that were spiraling out of control. A counselor pointed out that I was clinging to heartache as a misguided way to stay connected to my son, but having that insight didn't help me move through the pain. Everything in the basement of my being needed to come up and be either healed or tossed out. Many times I felt as if the hurt would never end, but gradually I began to make peace with my shadow side—the parts of myself I had tried to hide or deny.

One of my first steps forward was reading the book *Healing Your Aloneness* by Erika J. Chopich and Margaret Paul, which showed me how to start healing my relationship with my inner child. I also confided to a few friends that I felt like I had a big black hole in my gut, and one urged me to join a support group. There I heard other women speak with honesty about their struggles and, seeing them move through their suffering, felt hope that I, too, would rise out of the darkness.

It took years, but I'm whole now. One thing I've discovered is that all fear is a fear of feelings. And while feeling everything is hard, what's harder is missing the being human part by not feeling. I also learned that healing happens. You can get to a point where you're not only healed but actually have to make an effort to remember past misery. Figuring out what lessons you have learned from a difficult experience is helpful but doesn't fully release you from pain. Only love can do that. Through it all, you can learn to trust in yourself. More importantly, you can learn to rely on the power of something greater than yourself working through you. In facing the hurt, your Wise Woman can remind you, "You're being given painful experiences as gifts. Though sometimes the gifts are wrapped in sandpaper, you've got to go through them to grow through them. The more you accept and embrace these life lessons, the more mastery and grace you will enjoy."

Pema Chödrön, the American Buddhist nun and author of *When Things Fall Apart*, tells us that we actually need our pain. She writes: "To stay with that shakiness—to stay with a broken heart, with a rumbling stomach, with the feeling of hopelessness and wanting to get revenge—that is the path of true awakening. Sticking with that uncertainty, getting the knack of relaxing in the midst of chaos, learning not to panic—this is the spiritual path."[1] She explains that when you find yourself caught in extreme discomfort, the pain itself isn't the problem. If you can have a direct experience of that pain, it will be a great teacher for you, and you can survive it. If you stay with the pain and feel your way to the other side—you not only survive but become a more assured and aware version of yourself.

Understanding the Purpose of Pain

None of us would consciously choose to be in pain. Indeed, if you are hurting right now your mind may be flooded with such questions as: Why is this happening to me? How can I make it not hurt so much? Will this distress ever end? Many spiritual teachers tell us that painful events happen not to punish us because we're bad people but to help us master the life lessons we came here to learn. As Matt Kahn advises in his YouTube video *The Pain of Loss*, instead of insisting on "my way" we can learn to surrender in the face of upheaval and say, "Show me the way."[2]

If you wonder how a difficult situation you face could possibly be good for you, consider that it might be happening to:

- Redirect your life journey
- Teach you something you need to know
- Introduce you to someone who's important for you to meet

- Build an aspect of character that you'll need later
- Strengthen your ability to trust

Each of these objectives is transformative, making it worth the effort it takes to survive the challenges. Whatever the purpose may be for your pain, if you take the risk of confronting the hurt—whether this takes months, years, or decades—surviving it will feel like a miracle. You'll be more resilient and kinder, and you'll be of greater service to the world. You'll feel an intense desire to live, eager to start each day and surprised by how much energy you have. You'll have more to give, and giving won't drain you. The worry lines on your face will melt. By the smile on your lips, everyone will know you've been up to something a little mischievous. You'll catch a glimpse of yourself in the mirror and think, *Oh my, yes!*

Here's what else happens when you get through the big hurt. Not much will scare you. You'll no longer settle for second best. You won't twist yourself into knots to please other people. You'll feel your allies surrounding you, loving you, and helping you. You'll see other people through eyes of love. You'll emit a unique light, and in your presence others will recognize their own light. And you'll have conquered a fear that might otherwise have kept you from fulfilling your true potential.

Kahlil Gibran poignantly expressed this need for risk taking, despite the fear that may arise, to become more of who we are. In his poem "The River Cannot Go Back," he wrote: "It is said that before entering the sea, a river trembles with fear.…But there is no other way. The river cannot go back.… The river needs to take the risk of entering the ocean because only then will fear disappear, because that's where the river will know it's not about disappearing into the ocean, but of becoming the ocean."[3]

BREATHING SPACE

I enjoy feeling the flow of life.

I give myself permission to rest.

In my presence, others see their own light.

PRACTICE

Dare to Rest—Relaxation to Promote Focus and Quiet the Mind

This highly effective relaxation technique shared by Margaret Pittenger—a physical therapist and Feldenkrais practitioner known as a "miracle worker" for her ability to help people realign their bodies, avoid surgery, and live free from pain—will quickly intensify your ability to better focus, be calmer, and be kinder to loved ones and yourself.

- Lie with your hips supported in a 90/90 position, such as on the floor with your knees bent at a 90-degree angle and legs on a couch or coffee table, or on a bed with your legs on an ottoman or bolster. Make yourself warm and comfortable enough to begin letting go of tension.

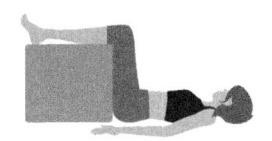

90/90 position

- Place both hands on your belly and feel the rhythm of your breath as you allow your belly to rise while you breathe in and fall while you breathe out. Relax for as long as possible on the exhalation.

- Focus on how your muscles respond to each inhalation and exhalation as your hands relay this information to your brain. While processing the information, your brain is building a better idea of how to interact with these muscles and ultimately create a neural pathway for this new way of being.

- Establish a rhythm of breathing in for 5 seconds and breathing out for 7 to 8 seconds. The prolonged exhalations will help you relax more completely.
- Continue this breathing pattern for 15 to 30 minutes.

Ordinarily, the most challenging part of relaxing is quieting the mind. Our minds are incessantly occupied. A fast-moving multitasker may not even understand that her mind doesn't have to be active all the time — that, on the contrary, it needs rest in order to organize all that she learns in a day. The body position for this practice helps calm the mind, due to three factors: the position of the hips, the position of the diaphragm muscle, and the chemical reaction produced in the brain when the hips and diaphragm relax. Normally, during the course of any day your brain, hips (psoas muscles), and diaphragm exchange chemical information you might think of as "backyard over-the-fence gossip." Any time your hips are overactive, for instance, they will seek more energy by producing chemicals in the area where the psoas muscles attach to the spine. Your psoas are emotional muscles, as is your diaphragm — attached to your spine in the same area — and your brain, reacting to every thought and emotion that runs through your head. The fervent "chatter" can easily prove stressful; but when you move into the 90/90 position, the relaxation of your hips and diaphragm can help stabilize the chemical reaction produced in your brain, thereby calming your mind.

This practice can not only help you relax, but it can do so quickly if you immerse yourself in it for 15 to 30 minutes daily for 3 consecutive days. Unlike most relaxation methods, which can take months to produce a positive outcome, "Dare to Rest" usually delivers results within days. By then, just lying in this position invites your body to relax and your mind to become quiet. The more you do this practice, the more support your body will deliver, in every way it can. And you will likely discover, as did Dutch author Etty Hillesum, who was killed in Auschwitz at age twenty-nine, that "sometimes the most important thing in a whole day is the rest we take between two deep breaths."[4]

Why are you so determined to keep your wild silently inside you? Let it breathe. Give it a voice. Let it roll out of you on the wide open waves. Set it free.

~Jeanette LeBlanc

CHAPTER 6

Embracing the Wildness Within

*Reconnecting with Nature
and the Sacred Power of Your Body and Voice*

During my childhood, I experienced a dramatic expression of inner wildness and freedom that has continued to remind me of an important truth. When I was three years old, a big black bull lived in the field behind our apartment. Every morning I pulled a small wooden chair over to a chest of drawers in my bedroom so I could climb up and peek out the window into his fenced pasture. Now and then I would catch a glimpse of that beast with his shaggy head hanging down, munching on grass, and, mesmerized by the sight of him, I would stare until my mother whisked me off the dresser into her arms, asking, "Are you watching that bull again?"

One summer day, dressed in a seersucker romper, I ventured off our front porch into the strip of yard that separated our apartment from the bull's pasture. I looked at the cloudless blue sky framing his massive body and big curved horns. His enormous head turned so he could gaze at me, his glistening nostrils flaring with each breath. I don't know how long we stood there watching each other. I only know that everything changed the moment he charged toward the fence, a few strands of silver cable between me and this fascinating, frightening creature. I gasped when the barbed wire squealed, his chest hitting metal with a violent force. Magnetized by some mix of awe and fear, I couldn't look away. I was afraid of the bull yet strangely excited by his power. With his wet, black eyes fixed on mine, I knew that in some sense he was speaking to me heart to heart—wild calling to wild—saying: "It may look like I'm trapped, but I'm still a wild bull. Never forget, your essence cannot be contained."

This message made no sense to me as a child. But while recalling the scene later in life, I believed the bull was instructing me to see that no matter what circumstances I faced, my essence could remain free. "One does not meet oneself," the naturalist Loren Eiseley has written, "until one catches the reflection from an eye other than human."[1]

Many of us living in the modern world have forgotten our roots in nature, the sweet song of the sunset, the creative flow and mystery of life. As a result, we've forgotten the sacred potency of our human bodies and voices, and even our hearts. We may feel confined by our job, boredom, the expectations of others, or the life we've settled for. Yet, as the bull's message suggests, even when feeling fenced in we can connect with our untamed self.

Our connection to nature is profound and essential for our well-being. As humans, each of us embodies all the elements—earth, water, wind, and fire. Our bodies are like earth; our bones are like her boulders. Our blood courses through us much as rivers flow to the ocean. Our breath is the air and our spirit the fire. Through this connection to Mother Earth and her elements, we become charged with her power and energy. As we tap into the cycles of nature, we return to a deep reverence for ourselves and all life. Even in our Wise Woman years we can summon our Maiden energy to rediscover our essential nature and refresh ourselves for the years ahead.

Encountering the Wildness Within

When we befriend our Maiden self, we give ourselves permission to take chances, explore, and try new things, as exemplified by a friend in her late thirties who shared memories from her early twenties, before she had begun shouldering the responsibilities of raising children and embarking on a career: "At the time, I traveled all over the world and felt powerful because I didn't think I had to know what I was doing yet. I was still figuring out my life and felt I could create what I wanted it to be. I didn't need a lot because I could sleep on a floor and make do with whatever meals I put together. I enjoyed the risk aspects, too. I found I could rely on help from other people, and I trusted in the goodness of life. All this was partly an outcome of my privileged childhood and partly who I was.

"During one of those summers, I went to Namibia by myself to study. I felt that people would help me and I'd be fine. The day I left Africa I was in line to fly home, but I hadn't thought to bring my boarding pass and only had a receipt from my previous flight. The check-in assistant said, 'This is not a boarding pass.' Unabashed, I dissolved into tears. The airlines eventually let me on the plane without the proper document. Looking back, I'm sure some of the wildness I felt had to do with not knowing that I was supposed to be embarrassed about things I hadn't yet figured out. I've since heard that the word *shame* is an acronym for 'should have already mastered everything.' And I've come to regard *should* as a violent word because it sets up an expectation that the way I am or something I do isn't okay. So now when encountering the unknown, rather than try to hide my ignorance, I say, 'I have no idea how this is supposed to work,' and I remind myself,

'It's okay for me not to know.' Being okay with not knowing things opens me to the possibility of being supported by others and trusting that I will be guided."

My own transformative encounter with the unknown came in my late fifties during a women's retreat led by Edwene Gaines, a dynamic spiritual teacher in her eighties. On the final day of the event, she prepared us for an initiation ceremony that would take place at sunset. Each activity was focused on the moment when we would confront our fears, the instant of deciding whether we had the courage to overcome them and walk barefoot across a ritual fire. In the morning, we listened to the song "Standing Outside the Fire" by Garth Brooks and were captivated by its concluding lyrics:

> *Life is not tried, it is merely survived*
> *If you're standing outside the fire.*

In the afternoon, we accepted an invitation to stand in a circle, name our fears, and express our desire to overcome them. As each woman spoke of her big dreams and the inner thoughts blocking her from actualizing them—I'm too old, people will judge me, I'll go bankrupt, I'm not smart enough—the other women listened, silently honoring her intention to take the next steps forward on her personal journey.

At sunset, we walked in silence along a path through the trees to a meadow. Approaching a stack of freshly split firewood, each woman lifted one log to represent her fears and fed it to the bonfire. The sun slipped behind the trees bordering the meadow, deepening the shadows in the forest, and purple irises stood in silent witness, waving in the gentle breeze alongside a gurgling creek. I heard the slap of bare feet on the cool, red clay as I followed the other women circling the ritual fire of our initiation ceremony. The feathers woven into our hair danced in the wind, and our beads and bracelets jingled softly in the night air as we swayed in rhythm to our chant:

Release your mind
See what you find
Bring it back home to your people.

With a shiver up my back, I had the sense that indigenous grandmothers' spirits were standing watch, silently blessing our presence and our courage.

As we circled the flames, quietly connecting with our higher guidance, we were advised to ask ourselves three questions: Can I walk on fire tonight and not be burned? Do I want to? Is it mine to do? A "yes" reply to all three questions indicated that we could walk on fire that night without injury.

I asked for guidance and received this message: "Yes, you are ready to walk on fire tonight and not be burned." As I watched each woman cross the wide expanse of glowing coals, I felt my resolve grow stronger. Each of us was calling on our courage to walk this path—for ourselves, for one another, and for all women.

When it was my turn to step forward, Edwene stood steadfast on my right, dressed head to toe in white and shimmering in the darkness like an angel. I took her hand and felt the pulse of love between us. I was tempted to look at my bare feet, but instead I glanced forward and saw two women waiting at the other end of the pathway to receive me. I heard an inner voice say, *Take the first step with an intention to be on the other side,* and so I did.

I don't recall any sensation of heat as I walked on the fiery embers. Rather, it felt like moving across a cushion of air until I reached the other side, where the two waiting women grasped my arms and guided me to step into a shallow pool of water. I felt taller, and my heart was wide open. I knew I wasn't the same woman who had come through the forest an hour earlier. Since that night I've been carrying a new awareness: *Now that I've walked on fire, I know I can do anything.* This experience taught me two crucial lessons—when you decide to face your fear, you recognize that you are already a fire walker, and when you honor your body's wisdom and your intuition, the wild woman within mirrors to you the true essence of who you are.

The Wisdom of Inner Wildness

As we enter the Wise Woman phase of life, many of us feel a call to "rise up," shaking us to our core. This is our Maiden self imploring us to shrug off our accumulated layers of social programming, mind-numbing beliefs, and outdated habits. We may have spent so many years conforming to the expectations of others that we're exhausted, disappointed, and restless. We feel unseen and unknown instead of fulfilled by engaging our inner wildness and being who we truly are.

And yet, when a woman is living a "fine" life with a partner who loves the version of her that supports their lifestyle, she can feel tremendous guilt at merely the thought of prioritizing her own goals and happiness. After all, she has a life that women are taught to be grateful for. So she tries to discount her desires and do what her conditioning tells her is expected. But a voice inside keeps insisting: *I want to be wild. I want to live according to the reality I imagine.*

Embracing the Wildness Within

Facing fear and taking a risk such as this unleashes immense energy. In the nineteenth century, when buffalo roaming the plains of North America saw dark clouds on the horizon, the herd would run as fast as they could toward the darkness, instinctively knowing this was the quickest way through the storm.[2] It's scary to act in a manner that we know will upset others, especially when we've been told our role is to keep the peace no matter what. And there can be a price to pay for following our core instincts. But there is a bigger price to pay if we abandon ourselves.

Of course, not all women need to leave their marriages or trek through the Himalayas to be who they truly are. Wherever you are in daily life, you can face your fear and move forward, each step further awakening your courage and drawing you closer to your essence. Moving forward often means speaking your truth, even when incidents threaten to silence your inner knowing. For example, you can tell someone who has bullied you that their behavior was hurtful and unnecessary. You can tell your boss you won't tolerate his demeaning behavior. You can tell your business partner that you know she lied. You can tell your husband that you're no longer willing to settle for the dry crumbs of your marriage.

The Power of Speaking Up

In speaking our truth, we give birth to the reality we envision. Interestingly, a woman's body is designed with two resonance chambers—the throat and the womb. Viewed from above, the structure of the larynx (voice box)[3] is remarkably similar to the bone formation of the pelvis (crucible of the womb).[4] On a physical as well as metaphoric level, both these spaces are centers for creation. The oracle at Delphi in ancient Greece, priestesses who were consulted on all matters of state importance, would squat over a crevice in the ground to receive wisdom directly into their wombs and were said to have the gift of "honey-voiced singing."[5]

Having an open flow of energy between heart, throat, and head allows us to hear inner guidance, not in words but in vibration and the feeling of being centered and grounded. An open flow of energy in the throat creates a bridge between the heart and head, allowing us to express what is authentically emerging from our hearts. When the throat is closed, messages from the heart become stifled by the critical inner voice, which complains, judges, and second-guesses. An effective way to open your throat is by writing down your fears, resentments, and jealousies and then taking a walk to let the feelings move through you. Humming and singing also help move energy through the throat.

A common cause for obstruction in the flow of energy through women's throats, stopping them from speaking their truth, is a conditioned belief in their own unworthiness. Those filled with big feelings were told they were "too much." Those who sensed what animals felt and saw things grownups couldn't see were called "odd." Those harboring ambitious views of their futures were labeled "unrealistic." In my case, what I witnessed around me as a young child was so out of sync with what I felt inside that I concluded there was something wrong with me. In response, I told myself to stay hidden and I started numbing myself with food, a habit that led to a full-blown eating disorder in my thirties.

If you wonder whether you harbor feelings of unworthiness, notice how you feel when someone says you're selfish. Women have been taught that the highest compliment is being told they're selfless, which basically means they're lacking a self. We've been damaged by such lies, but as we learn to embrace our inner essence and listen to our Maiden and Wise Woman, we gain better perspective and experience our inherent worthiness. The the more we reevaluate what we've been taught, what we've read, and what we've believed about ourselves, the better we become at detecting such lies and replacing them with what we know to be true. Welcoming the gifts of our Maiden and Wise Woman, we stop caring so intently about the opinions of others, find our voices, and begin speaking up.

A friend in her late forties described how she reclaimed her voice during menopause: "Going forward, I got clear that if something isn't completely aligned, doesn't fully light me up, and I don't get to be a thousand percent unapologetically myself in it, then it's not meant to be. I speak up now and say I don't want it. Full stop. I finally realized that this is not selfish — it's self-love."

The Power of Connecting to Natural Resources

The stress of daily life often sends us into fight, flight, or freeze mode; interacting with natural resources, however, shifts us into rest-and-digest mode, linking us to comparable resources within our own bodies and thereby increasing our sense of security and well-being. To cultivate an immediate connection with natural resources that will nourish and enliven you, interact often with the elements. For some women, it is grounding to have their feet on soil, whether in a forest or their front yard. For others, proximity to flowing water or a certain plant or tree awakens a connection to nature. Interacting with the elements can be as simple as running your hands through a bowl of sand or listening to birdsong.

Being in nature, even feeling in tune with nature, transforms us. Life forces we sense in the natural world—while looking at a flower with soft fascination, for example, or feeling a cool breeze on our skin—can calm us enough to tell ourselves we're safe. Similarly, a sudden flash of lightning can make us aware that we, too, are alive with energy. Simply put, while absorbed in nature we are not the same beings as when we're ensconced in a sterile office building. Dr. Joanna Macy, a renowned teacher of deep ecology who has devoted her life to helping humanity connect to its roots, describes the aliveness we feel and the sustenance we receive from interacting with nature: "To be alive in this beautiful, self-organizing universe—to participate in the dance of life with senses to perceive it, lungs that breathe it, organs that draw nourishment from it—is a wonder beyond words."[6]

My friend Lindsey, a birth doula and eco-activist who, inspired by Macy's work, offers outdoor retreats focused on healing through nature, states: "Joanna Macy helped me see that I belong to the world. So if I go to a place that's been strip-mined or logged, or if I see an animal that's been hit by a car, the impulse in me to bring healing to that situation doesn't just come from me. It comes from a very real relationship to that place or that being. I learned the term *bodhichitta* heart—the impulse and the ability to respond to what's wounded, based on the idea that we are connected to every living thing. When I can see not only the whole forest but myself as part of the whole forest, then I can actually be resourced—enlivened and strengthened—by it and also see myself in the proper scale. As a child, I was taught to dismiss my intuitive knowing. I was told that if you feel something in your body, you should immediately start to analyze it because unless it's measurable and concrete it cannot be trusted. Now I realize that's only one way to view the world. A more visceral and direct way is to just sit with it, be in sync with it, and trust the knowing that comes. Intuitive knowing takes practice, and trusting it requires me to be around people who support me in doing so, because it's still fragile."

Currently, many of us feel we're giving birth to new ways of being in relationship with others and the earth. Dr. Macy calls this shift from the industrial growth society to a life-sustaining civilization the "Great Turning" and considers it the essential transformation of our time.[7] To prepare for this shift, we need to cultivate awareness on three levels, beginning with the recognition that we're part of the natural world and our lives depend on it. We also need to become skilled at heeding the messages our bodies consistently send—such as the realization that we're slouching in our chair because we've been sitting all morning or our stomach is growling because we're hungry. And we must practice bringing awareness to our actions so they become our default in crisis situations. For example, if we practice not snapping at loved ones when we're tired, the resulting patience will be our future "go-to" behavior in stressful situations.

An aware, alert mindfulness of our body's wisdom and our actions operates as a gentle daily reminder that we are responsible for our own serenity. By following our hearts with steadfast courage and devotion to our own truth and by sustaining ourselves through connections to natural resources, we can know the freedom of living as sovereign beings. The most nurturing thing a woman can do is know herself, trust herself, and pursue what she wants without apology. When we grant ourselves permission to embrace our inner wildness and live as our freest selves, we automatically grant permission to everyone around us to do the same.

BREATHING SPACE

I breathe and feel
my connection to every living thing.

As I appreciate Mother Earth,
she is nourished by my love.

Today my Maiden helps me feel
the wildness moving in my body.

PRACTICE

Connecting with Your Wild Inner Nature

The best way to connect with your wild inner nature is by returning to the wild in nature. If you have been feeling ungrounded, overwhelmed, or preoccupied with time management, productivity, and efficiency—sometimes carving out thirty minutes for a run outdoors but never looking at the treetops or pausing to rest your bare feet on the earth—remind yourself that the wildlife around you remains patient, waiting for you to remember that you belong to nature. The only provisions needed for your return to the wild are a recognition that you carry within you your untamed self, in the form of a young child with her instinctual nature still intact, and that you wish to release her from captivity and deepen your relationship with her.

To do so, take the following five steps:

- Arrange a time and place for a sense walk in nature, a trek during which you will tune in to your senses. Clear at least 2 hours for this activity, enough time for you to transition from a mental to a sensory orientation to your surroundings, from intellect to intuition, doing to being. Make sure the place you choose is more densely populated with animal and plant life than human life, because then you will more likely experience the trees, birds, and other creatures communicating with you and inviting you into their world.

- Go to your chosen place, stand still, and take a few breaths deep into your belly, relaxing your jaw and shoulders. Then set an intention to remain present to your immediate experiences. Next, visualize a threshold beyond which lies the natural environment you wish to explore. Introduce yourself; ask for permission to enter; and once you have received consent to step over the threshold, begin walking, guided by your intuition, into this landscape.

- Continuing on your walk, engage with the landscape through each of your senses. Listen closely to the sounds around you. Slow your pace and feel your feet touching the ground; lightly move your hands across the bark of a nearby tree, feeling its texture and temperature against your skin — or if you are at the shore, explore the sand, water, and shells through touch. Smell the flowers and taste the air. Allow your eyes to caress the sky. Take in the colors and patterns of the space around you, including contrasts between its light and darkness. Practice listening, touching, smelling, tasting, and seeing in sequence until you feel a deep resonance with this place.

- Remembering yourself as a young girl viewing the world through eyes of wonder, search for the presence of your inner child within you. When you find her, free her of any shackles imposed during her decades of confinement and let her out to play. For guidance in releasing her, follow your intuition. Perhaps take your shoes off and wiggle your toes in the sand, or walk barefoot in the creek bed. Or sing to the birds, listening for them to sing back. Or go off trail, sit on a fallen tree, and watch the forest come alive. When you feel her presence, look delightedly into the faces of nearby flowers. Write down the poetry flowing from your heart. Then take a deep breath and acknowledge that you are once again wild and free.

- Close by making an offering of gratitude from your heart to the earth. A prayer, a song, or a treasured leaf or shell will more than suffice. As you leave this wild place, feel the wildness moving in your body and remind yourself that you belong to the earth and she belongs to you.

After completing a sense walk, many women feel not only in touch with their wildness but also more centered and grounded. No longer agitated or irritable, they are able to gain fresh perspective on matters related to their health, relationships, or direction in life. Some return to their special place whenever they feel a need to tap back into their essence in a space where their wildness can breathe. Invariably, they emerge empowered and refreshed.

*What if desire wasn't an urge to be tamed
but a beacon of truth to be followed?*

~Danielle LaPorte

CHAPTER 7

Joygasms Galore

Feeling More Sensual, Sexy, and Happy

As women age, many, like my friend Jill, worry that loss of sexual desire is inevitable. I invited her to come talk with me about an issue that was troubling her. We kicked off our shoes and settled into lounge chairs on the screen porch. The fragrance of roses mingled with the sound of the wind chimes. Jill took a sip of iced tea and looked down, embarrassed. She was entering perimenopause and concerned about the changes in her periods, but she was mainly nervous because while making love with her partner Alex, her sexual desire seemed to be fading. Although sex had been a beautiful part of Jill's relationship with Alex for ten years, which she described as loving and romantic, now she was having to work harder to become aroused. She didn't want him to feel she was losing interest in him or that he wasn't doing a good job. She confided, "I've been overthinking it and getting distracted. Then I feel self-conscious, which is definitely a buzzkill. I'm afraid we might lose what we've had." Because her mind was running the show and her fear made her anxious, it was hard for her to surrender to the pleasure she had enjoyed with Alex in the past.

When we get older we may assume changes in our bodies indicate we must give up having sensual and sexual pleasure in our lives. But, contrary to the prevailing narrative, we do not have to forfeit such pleasure as we age. In fact, as psychotherapist and author Esther Perel affirms, "Passion is about a quality of aliveness. It's about the permission to feel good."[1] When we feel vibrant and energized, life becomes orgasmic. Even though it wasn't true for me before menopause, now "joygasms"—spiritual, creative, emotional, and physical—happen frequently. Based on conversations I've had with female friends and clients, I believe that we all want this exuberant response to life and that it can emerge once we become aware of what is standing in our way.

Getting Naked—Valuing Your Sexual Self

Not valuing our sexual selves can undermine our physical and emotional well-being and ultimately our potential for fulfillment in life. The medical view in the mid-nineteenth century was that women did not have organs of sexual pleasure. In his widely quoted book of advice for men, Dr. William Acton stated: "The majority of women (happily for them) are not very much troubled with sexual feelings of any kind."[2] But the truth is that women are designed to experience pleasure, and it's our birthright to enjoy sensual satisfaction. In fact, it costs us dearly when we don't value our sexual selves, as some measure of breakdown happens at work, at home, in our relationships, and with our emotional and physical well-being when we're not satisfied and self-expressed sexually.

Since this is so, why do we have trouble pursuing or feeling sensual satisfaction, and why do we still have a hard time talking about female sexuality and pleasure? For one thing, we often feel conflict between our bodies' needs and society's expectations. We're frequently told to keep our desires private or suppress them, while every cell in our bodies is praying that we'll begin to understand and celebrate our sexual selves. At such times we can call on our inner Maiden and Queen for help.

The obstacles blocking us from feeling sensual and sexual pleasure include fears of:

- Not being enough
- Hurting our partner
- Not being loved for who we are
- Being rejected based on how we look
- Feeling vulnerable

It takes considerable courage to face such fears. But when we do we come to truly accept ourselves, knowing we're actually unlimited, empowered beings capable of far more than we've been told.

We can start overcoming the fears impeding our experience of sensual and sexual pleasure by recognizing that we've been sold a bill of goods telling us we aren't lovable or that someone's going to love us not for who we are but for how we look. Although one way to express love is through the body, people generally do not love others based on the appearance of body parts. You can explore this with your partner by cultivating the willingness to love each other without reservation as a daily practice. Although you may fear that your partner will reject you or that you might feel embarrassed, focus on the well-being of your beloved, asking yourself: "Am I wishing my partner well or not?" Then imagine that good things could happen when you risk opening your heart and refuse to take offense at your partner's actions.

Joygasmic Girl Talk

Why is women's pleasure so mysterious? As author Eve Ensler comments in *The Vagina Monologues*: "It would be years before I learned that females possessed the only organ in the human body with no function other than to feel pleasure."[3] Honestly, how many women know what reliably brings them to a satisfying orgasm? Most of us were not given sufficient guidance on women's pleasure, and it's hard to find accurate information about this topic since the ways women are sexually gratified vary and the subject is shrouded by myths, opinions, and rumors, especially in pop culture. However, regardless of your age or situation, if you aren't in a sexual relationship with a partner, if your partner's sexual desire is less than yours, or if you're ready to learn more about what feels good, now is a perfect time to become more familiar with your body and your most intimate desires.

A good way to start is by learning about some of the ways you can pleasure yourself. In conversing with women about their erogenous experiences, I'm often reminded that the power to feel good is literally in our hands.

Enjoying Orgasms

An orgasm is first perceived in the brain, which then sends electrical signals to the genitals, triggering an intensely pleasurable spasm of the pelvic floor muscles that can last ten to fifteen seconds or longer.[4] Research from Indiana University shows that orgasms have numerous physical benefits in addition to emotional ones. They boost the immune system and help fight depression. They are one of the most effective ways of keeping pelvic floor muscles strong and toned, which can help prevent urinary incontinence. Additionally, the more orgasms you have the easier it will be for you to orgasm in the future.[5]

Many women don't have what is conventionally described as orgasms, yet they still have fulfilling sex lives. Most feel liberated upon realizing they don't need to live up to someone else's concept of what their sexual pleasure should be. Others feel they are missing out on something important and want to experience the gratification of orgasmic release. And some women, frightened of losing control over their bodies, find it difficult to relax fully enough to have orgasms.

To explore what feels best, start by experimenting with yourself, free from expectations. After finding a private place where you will not be disturbed, locate areas of your body that give you the most pleasure when touched. Relax and focus on stimulating those areas with your fingers, using a small amount of lubricant so they move more smoothly without irritating your skin. Any water-based lubricant is fine but not oil, Vaseline, or anything scented as these products can irritate your skin and lead to yeast infections.[6]

The types of hand stimulation that many women enjoy are strokes on the vulva (outer lips of the vagina), stroking or rubbing in and around the mouth of the vagina, and especially stroking or rubbing the clitoris, either its shaft or its tip. You might like long strokes over these areas, or perhaps short, quick touches in a circular motion that get faster as you become more aroused. Your leg muscles may get tense, which can be part of the process. Try different ways of touching various areas, with diverse pressures and speeds. Control how far you go each time you pleasure yourself, building more tension and sensation on every occasion. Focus on what is enjoyable to you, and let a sense of playfulness move you. When you find something that feels good, continue touching yourself that way. If it stops feeling good, try another type of touch. Know that what feels best can change as you move from the Maiden to the Queen to the Wise Woman stage of life.

Using Personal Intimate Devices

Research reveals that only 18 percent of women have orgasms from penetration alone, compared to 73 percent who have orgasms when clitoral stimulation is added. These orgasms are shown to be more frequent and more pleasurable.[7] Based on these findings, if you aren't able to have an orgasm from hand stimulation or your hand gets tired, you may want to use a vibrator, a dildo, or both. This is also a good alternative if:

- You want to explore another way to become sexually aroused.
- You want to experience more than one orgasm.
- Your partner is tired, ill, not interested in sex when you are, or finished with sex before you are.
- You have arthritis in your hands.

If vibrators are new territory for you, choose one with variable intensities. A budget-friendly option is to use the pulsing stream of water from a removable shower head. Products for internal stimulation come in a surprising variety of sizes, materials, colors, and textures. If you're not sure how to pick the right one, try a variety of them and choose a few favorites. (See pages 170 and 171 at the end of this book for discreet shopping recommendations.)

Also try different positions. Lying on your back might work well, or sitting, balancing on hands and knees, or even standing up. Be creative and pay attention to your sensations in different positions and while using varying intensities of stimulation. Keep experimenting until you find something you like.

In addition, let yourself explore fantasies. Erotic books, audios, or movies can help arouse your imagination. Play with your breath as well, taking long, deep breaths to slow things down or short, panting ones to heighten arousal. Knowing what feels good to you is the ultimate in independence.

One woman I interviewed shared her delight in experimenting with various tools and techniques: "It wasn't until my late forties, when divorced from my former husband, that I explored my sexuality more deeply. One man liked that I brought in vibrators and other toys because he enjoyed seeing me having pleasure. He said it helped him learn what I liked and took the pressure off him to have an erection or to perform. Another man didn't like it at all. So at first I responded, 'Well, okay, we don't have to use them.' But eventually I said, 'Forget that! If you don't want these in the bed, then you don't really care about my pleasure.' Not until I approached age fifty did I realize I could reach a more intense level of orgasm with a partner and stay there."

Remember, your enjoyment of sensual play can increase over your lifetime, with new experiences bringing a sense of surprise and delight. So don't ever think you're too old to explore self-pleasuring, even if you're used to having a sexual partner or haven't enjoyed sexual pleasure in a long time.

Telling Your Partner What You Like in Bed
Silent sex, the kind we see in movies, doesn't work very well. Although a partner may think they know exactly what a woman

likes, or the woman may expect her partner to read her mind, every woman is different and no particular move works every time. It is preferable to show or tell your partner what you like. Your partner will thank you for not expecting them to be a mind reader. Self-pleasure is the best way to learn what you like so that you can teach your partner the most effective techniques. In fact, many women find it easier to have an orgasm with a partner after discovering what works solo. If you determine that a vibrator works well for you, try using it on your partner—both men and women enjoy the sensations—and demonstrating what you enjoy by including it in your sex play.

Finding Support
If you want savvy girlfriends willing to share confidential insights about their sex lives and techniques, one resource is an affordable private-membership website called OMGYes. There, in videos of women ages eighteen to ninety-five talking about their experiences, you'll find advice and methods for enhancing your sexual pleasure. The techniques are based on research involving more than twenty thousand women and are categorized so you (and your partner) can learn how sexual pleasure differs for each woman.

When interviewed on a podcast for Webby award winners in 2017, the founders of OMGYes, Lydia Daniller and Rob Perkins, said they created this website to normalize conversations on intimacy, stating: "We want people to see pleasure the same way they see cooking. If you read a cookbook, it doesn't mean you're a bad cook and need help. It means you're probably a good cook, and you're curious and want to explore and try new recipes."[8]

Sex for the Soul

Techniques are valuable, but sex is most rewarding when we venture beyond the mechanics involved. Toward that end, a helpful audiobook is *Tantra: Sex for the Soul* by Niyaso Carter, a guide for creating sexual awareness based on the ability to be transparent with another person.[9] Tantra is commonly misunderstood to be a series of difficult, esoteric sexual positions. But to Carter it's about the practice of being real with someone. We spend vast amounts of time building our careers, making money, and taking care of other people, but usually not much time making love or being transparent with our significant other. And the time we do spend often becomes a little humdrum if we've been with that person for a while, sometimes making us think our sex drive is disappearing.

However, it doesn't matter how many years we've been with a partner as long as we're willing to start fresh with a different point of view, which Carter's insights provide. Particularly enjoyable are her partner exercises, starting with eye-gazing and breathing together, then progressing to energy touch and genital massage. Another benefit is that this material, which Carter wrote to increase the potential of love on the planet, reframes the idea of making love from an activity in which partners satisfy each other sexually to one in which they actively express love by engaging their imaginations, playfulness, and curiosity.

Today, the dynamic between intimate partners is shifting from contractual love to unconditional love, from striving to fit the other person's idea of who you should be to viewing lovemaking as a practice of bringing love to its highest potential. In this type of intimacy, women and men feel honored and safe, and thus free to fully let go and enjoy themselves. Being loved for who you are as you show up relaxed and natural is being loved for who you are at your core.

Another interesting thing about this type of intimacy is that the sex is hot. The energy you bring to your lovemaking will intensify if it is based on acceptance and the willingness to see and be seen, touch and be touched, love and be loved, resulting in a cherished experience that will enrich all areas of your life. What's more, you don't need to have a partner to explore this type of lovemaking. *Tantra: Sex for the Soul* includes ways of working with your own energies.

Life as a Sensual Feast

When we embrace pleasure, life becomes a sensual feast regardless of our age. We don't have to buy in to the nonsense that older women are not sexy or that after menopause they can't enjoy pleasure. According to third-century Greek author Athenaeus, Cleopatra covered the floor of her bedroom with a thick, silken layer of rose petals and sprinkled rose water between her sheets to enhance her charms as a seductive temptress.[10] Whatever our age, we can always call on our inner Maiden to bring us back to the wonder of being in a body. Aging doesn't have to mean contracting. We can vow: "I'm aging, and I'm expanding my mental capacity, my physical health, and my ability to experience pleasure. I'm expanding my imagination, my creativity, and my heart's capacity for love."

Embracing sensual pleasure is a potent part of accepting and loving ourselves. Toward that end, be sure to cultivate awareness of what you are doing with your energy and how sexy you feel. It starts with your relationship with yourself and how you show up for yourself, including how you take care of your body, how you honor it, and whether the clothes you wear make you feel frumpy or self-confident. In this way, you can discover how to feed your inner fire.

If you're not already turning yourself on to life, now is the time to begin. Call on the creativity of your Maiden to give you a "feel good" permission slip. Every part of your day can be a mini pleasure ritual, from wearing a plush robe and cozy slippers to smoothing a creamy lotion over your face, neck, and legs. Think of yourself as a two-year-old who greets life through her senses by touching, tasting, smelling, and getting messy as she savors the delights that give life sweetness.

Experiencing pleasure can be especially advantageous if your busy, overscheduled life is keeping you agitated. At such times you need more oxytocin, the pleasure hormone, to balance the stress hormone (cortisol) your body is producing. Fortunately, your body secretes oxytocin during many enjoyable activities, such as hugging, laughing, petting animals, hanging out with friends, practicing yoga, breathing deeply, performing random acts of kindness, meditating, enjoying massages or sex, or listening to music. You just need to remind yourself: oxytocin over cortisol, fun over stress. The more fun you have, the better you'll feel and the more passion your actions will reflect, whether you are writing a postcard, stirring a pot of soup, walking your dog, or making love.

Although we've been taught that it's more virtuous to give than receive, welcoming pleasure—starting with small treats—helps us soften into more allowing, more receiving. When we accept life's indulgences, we become more generous, love ourselves more, and beam more love to others.

When you learn to embrace the pleasure you were born to enjoy, you will:

- See your body as beautiful and worthy of appreciation at any age.
- Trade overwhelm and obligation for passion and ease.
- Create your own "pleasure map" for every part of your life.
- Inspire other women by modeling self-celebration instead of self-denial.

Nurturing the ability to receive pleasure will also make you ultramagnetic. As a result, you're likely to become the happy recipient of other benefits, like fresh flowers delivered to your door, funding to launch a project, a new job offer, an upgrade to first class, or imaginative ideas when you least expect them.

Orgasmic energy literally creates life, the cocreative process in which we are engaged. Regardless of what you've been conditioned to believe, you are worthy of having this energy course through your body, mind, and heart.

Sexual Sovereignty—The Surprising Gift of the Wise Woman Phase

Counter to the messages we hear in our culture, as we enter the Wise Woman phase our sexual pleasure can be greater than at any previous age and can remain so into our sixties, seventies, and beyond. As Kelly, a woman I interviewed, told me with a bright smile, "I've had a good sex life with my husband for thirty years, but I'm surprised to discover it's gotten even better after menopause!"

Like Kelly, my sexual rebirth didn't begin until I was postmenopausal, in my early fifties. Before menopause, sex was good and I enjoyed orgasms, though I let my male partner run the show. I grew up at a time when information about women's bodies and sex was kept secret, and I never learned how to give myself pleasure. Scrupulously conditioned to put the man's needs first, I focused entirely on making sure he desired me and was satisfied, with my pleasure an afterthought, if I considered it at all. I didn't like my body and felt disconnected from it. I was uncomfortable being "seen" in every way, preferring to have sex in the dark and keep a protective emotional cage around my heart.

Only later did I sense there was something wonderful on the other side of my fears, an acceptance of myself beyond anything I had known. I read a book about extended massive orgasm. I bought a few sex toys and began having self-pleasure dates to discover what felt good. I hoped it would be fun, but at first I felt uncomfortable and embarrassed. Then over time I gained the ability to track and understand the subtle feedback my body was communicating. The hardest part was revealing all this to my husband. That was real intimacy, far beyond taking my clothes off and making love. He listened quietly, without trying to jump in and fix things, and I could see by the tenderness in his eyes that he empathized with me. When I finished talking, he held me in his arms. I felt ten pounds lighter and very relieved. The next day we had a conversation about what had surfaced, and we committed to practicing more transparency in our relationship going forward.

To cultivate a novel kind of intimacy, we had to feel safe and relaxed enough to play and take risks that felt fun-loving. Because we both worked from home, we set aside time each day for a "business meeting" to try new things, like dressing up for role play, exchanging fantasies, and receiving pleasure from the other without reciprocating. It was both scary and exciting, and our shared sense of humor kept us going. We saw our new experiences as a way to actively engage with life — which became a pathway to transformation for ourselves and our partnership. Even outside the bedroom we began smiling more and curling up on the sofa after dinner to celebrate the highlights of our day. A memory I will treasure until my last breath is when we made soul-touching love, tapping into a life force that felt more transcendent than I had ever imagined possible. Afterward I felt vibrantly alive as I pulled him to me, pressing our hearts together while an exchange of heat and light flashed between us. We call it the time we had a simultaneous "heartgasm."

Interestingly, many women I hear from in their Wise Woman phase of life have experienced spontaneous full-body orgasm in solitude, without touching themselves or entertaining sexual thoughts. One woman in her mid-fifties was driving on a busy freeway in Los Angeles and had to pull off at the nearest exit and park until the orgasm was over. A woman in her sixties was awakened in the middle of the night and taken on a wildly orgasmic ride in what she said felt like a waking dream. And a seventy-year-old woman was stopped in her tracks by a full-body orgasm while walking through her garden.

Some of the women mentioned that in these moments they felt kundalini energy. *Kundalini*, a Sanskrit word meaning "coiled one," refers to a form of primal energy spiraling upward from the base of the spine to the crown of the head.[10] Here's how a woman named Alice described her experience: "It started with a feeling like waves of energy coursing through my body, from my feet to the top of my head. Then a most unusual thing happened: moaning sounds began to come out of my throat, and my hips started to undulate. I felt like I was a giant anaconda writhing in pleasure. My back arched, and my pelvis thrust forward to receive. But receive what? Certainly not a man; I was alone. And it was more than sexual. Shivers shook my whole body. This extremely pleasant experience morphed into the sense of being filled with pure love. You might call it orgasmic, but that doesn't begin to describe what I felt. I can only describe it as love making love to itself."

Alice told me she had learned she could intentionally experience that euphoric state in certain settings: "First, I have to be relaxed, lying in a warm bath or on a comfortable bed. I set the intention to connect to a higher consciousness. I usually go into this space when I'm drifting off to sleep; it's like plugging into an electrical outlet and letting the current course through me. Then it's all there; I'm in orgasm throughout my body. To keep it going, I repeat a circular breath: I breathe into the base of my spine, let it flow up my back to the top of my head, then down the front of my body, around to the base of my spine, and up again. It's the breath of life."

Although not every woman in her Wise Woman years will enjoy a spontaneous full-body orgasm, simply being aware that these peaks of explosive joy can happen reminds us of how connected we are to the creative energy that flows through every living thing. Knowing that women in their Wise Woman phase are having such ecstatic experiences awakens us to the power of the feminine to spread love over the planet, radiating the supple and generous energy of life to all.

BREATHING SPACE

This is pleasure. I want more!

I enjoy feeling sensual and connected to my body.

Falling in love with myself and with life
is a choice I can make every day.

PRACTICE

Joygasm Bingo

To feel more vibrant and energized, and to experience your body as an instrument of radiance, play the self-pleasuring game of Joygasm Bingo. Just as standard bingo invites each player to mark the squares on their card that match those announced by the caller, Joygasm Bingo invites you, the sole player, to mark the squares on your card that describe sensual activities to which you have just treated yourself. While a few of them, such as "eye-gazed with my partner" or "showered together," are meant to be shared with a beloved, most are for enjoying alone—for increasing your willingness to surrender to pleasure or simply delighting in the creative energy associated with sexual pleasure.

To do this practice, choose a square on your card, then gather any "props" necessary for performing the activity described, such as an erotic movie, gourmet chocolate, or a silky camisole you may have been saving for a special occasion. Be indulgent; show your sexual self how much she is valued. Next, perform the action described. For some activities, you will want to give yourself the privacy of an indoor space before surrendering to the pleasure they arouse. Others, such as breathing fresh air or accepting a compliment, can be enjoyed outdoors or in public. While doing the activity, notice places of excitation in your body and feelings of expansiveness and tingling as you connect with it. Finally mark the square, indicating that the activity has been completed. After marking even one square on your card, consider yourself a Joygasm Bingo winner—a woman who has created time and space for savoring pleasure in her life!

As a winner at this practice, you will have also discovered that self-pleasuring is about infinitely more than the rush of endorphins. Surrendering to pleasure helps us develop a better understanding of our likes and dislikes, increased confidence to ask for what we want in life, a greater sense of self-worth, and a more optimistic perspective.

Joygasm BINGO

Breathed in fresh air	WORE SEXY UNDIES	Brushed Teeth NAKED, IN HEELS	LISTENED to My Body	Showered Together
jiggled & wiggled	Eye-gazed WITH MY partner	ACCEPTED A COMPLIMENT	Savored ONE YUMMY chocolate	RELISHED an erotic fantasy
Let myself CRY	Enjoyed a self-pleasure date	WOW!	Listened to Erotica	Indulged in a NEW LUBE
dessert ON ME... LITERALLY	Danced to a sensual playlist	WROTE MYSELF A love letter	PLAYED with VIBRATOR	Said THANK YOU to my body
Treated myself to an arousing movie	Affirmed: This is pleasure. I want more!	Wore a yoni egg	Adored my feet	Found my G-spot

Female friendships that work are relationships in which women help each other belong to themselves.

~Louise Bernikow

CHAPTER 8

Attracting an Angel Posse

The Transformative Power of Friendship, Community, and Creative Collaboration

Belonging to a group called Esther's Girls offered me and its other members profound lessons in how our Queen self can help us take advantage of supportive friendships and collaboration. Esther's Girls was conceived one August day in 1986 in the Gulf of Mexico. I had been bouncing around in the waves with four women friends when one, a professional dancer named Lyn, exclaimed, "Let's do back flips!" Although performing a back flip in the ocean using one arm while pinching your nose is generally impossible without gagging on gallons of salt water, we supported each other's backs and shouted encouragement until all five of us had done a full 360-degree flip. What happened next was so spontaneous that none of us had a chance to question its sanity. The woman closest to Lyn cried out, "Why don't we make up a swimming routine and perform it in the river at our dance camp next month?"

"Great idea!" everyone chimed in, as we wrapped our arms around one another, forming a circle and kicking in unison. Then, while the sun set over the ocean, we choreographed a routine faintly reminiscent of extravagant Hollywood aqua-musicals starring Esther Williams, the famous synchronized swimmer and movie star of the 1940s and 1950s. That routine marked the first of what was to become, by popular demand, an annual Esther's Girls event. Each subsequent year we devised a new theme for our presentation, which we practiced for weeks before performing it at our dance camp in the foothills of the Smoky Mountains.

I recall with fondness our sense of camaraderie one especially humid August day when we sweated profusely and giggled like schoolgirls while huddling around a tiny mirror in a musty cabin—five thirty-something women on a secret mission. Earlier we had squirmed into the 1950s-style bathing suits we had found at a small-town thrift store, among them a two-piece suit with polka dots, one with bright tropical flowers, and a sleek black number with buxom padding. Next, Martha passed around some bright red lipstick she had brought for us to share. Out of my backpack I pulled big ruffled silk flowers to clip into each woman's hair. Our arms and elbows bumped amiably while, sitting together on squeaky cots, we checked each other's makeup, adding a bit more blush and wiping lipstick off our front teeth. We then disguised ourselves in flowing bathrobes and pranced slowly, in our high heels, hand-in-hand down the gravel path leading to the river below for our performance.

Over the years, Esther's Girls grew to include many originally shy but later kickass women such as doctors, professors, mothers, therapists, business owners, and artists. We welcomed any woman who was brave enough to risk a few bruises and sore muscles while endeavoring to make each event unique. One year we staged our act in the gym, trying to execute a graceful waltz on roller skates while careening around the polished floor, grabbing each other's arms to keep from falling. Other years we performed Busby Berkeley–style tap dancing, African dances, and a routine to the country song

"Cleopatra, Queen of Denial" by Pam Tillis, dressed in short skirts, Egyptian-style bustier corsets, cowgirl boots, and big Stetson hats. During our final tenth anniversary performance, the grand finale, featuring the song "Good Vibrations" (with appropriate props), brought down the house.

Esther's Girls offered us invaluable support during that decade because we each knew the others in our circle would pick us up when we fell, celebrate with us when we flourished, and hold us when we were shattered. Together we weathered divorces, addiction, a child's life-threatening illness, and the death of one of our members in a tragic car accident. These women were an intimate circle of sisters I came to call my angel posse. For me, the group reflected the transformative power of friendship, community, and creative collaboration—a beacon that guided me to keep moving and growing.

Finding Friends Who See Your Essence

After the Esther's Girls club was dissolved, as a result of our increasingly busy lives, I became acutely aware of how important it was to have friends who could help us appreciate life's journey. I knew that when women are squeezed for time they typically first drop friendships and physical activity, even though these are proven happiness boosters and offer relief from feelings of overwhelm and separation. Many clients had told me that as they built careers, supported spouses and children, and devoted time to community causes and aging parents, they had no energy left to give themselves or their friends. What these women had lost was not only their friends but their connection to the Queen aspect of womanhood—the ability to get support and honor their own needs instead of focusing solely on accommodating those of others.

Following this realization, I started a local Radiant Wise Woman group to give women a safe place to connect and talk about aging with grace. When I surveyed the group about their greatest challenges with aging, most mentioned loneliness, isolation, and difficulty meeting people. Many had moved to Birmingham for jobs or family but had failed to find a close group of like-minded women friends. Most of those with grown children no longer shared a ready-made connection with other mothers through school and sports teams. Several reported that their co-workers had been their friends until the women retired and lost contact with them. Three shared the anguish of losing a spouse through divorce or death, describing their spouse as their only friend, which compounded their grief, leaving them no one to walk with through the pain. Other women had become isolated while grappling with a chronic illness, caring for a loved one round-the-clock, or coping with other challenges demanding their time and energy. For example, Vicky, a woman in her mid-fifties who struggled with fibromyalgia, stayed cocooned in her apartment for months, eating takeout food and binge-watching TV. Though earlier in life she had been athletic and accustomed to having all the energy she needed, now she felt too drained and ashamed to be around women friends.

At one of our gatherings, a woman named Rachel lingered as the others left the room. She quietly moved closer to me, her crystal blue eyes glistening with tears, and asked, "Lee, I'm feeling so lonely. Can I die from it?" The answer, unfortunately, is yes. Medical science has discovered that a lonely individual is significantly more likely to suffer an early death than someone intimately connected to at least one other person. Studies show that strong friendships boost immunity, reduce the risk of depression, and lengthen life—surprisingly, even more than losing weight or giving up smoking.[1] According to the groundbreaking Tend and Befriend study from UCLA, when women feel stressed and come together for mutual support they naturally secrete oxytocin, the same bonding hormone produced during breastfeeding and orgasm, which helps them feel calmer and more social.[2]

Regardless of how isolated you may be, there is a web of support available to you. Even if you have begun to drift from feeling "comfortable being alone" to feeling "uncomfortable being alone"—from enjoying solitude to contending with too much isolation—other women are ready to lend a hand when you reach out. For example, when Candace Pearl, recently divorced, found herself alone and facing a life-threatening health challenge, she rallied a few friends in a Facebook group that soon grew to over seventy women. After a full recovery, she founded Women Who Have Your Back, a network of women dedicated to providing hands-on support in their community.

Healing Wounds between Women

Cultural conditioning has taught us to believe that the resources available to us are limited. Therefore, we think we must compete, especially with other women, for men, jobs, recognition, and appreciation. As a result, many women experience disappointment, frustration, judgment, or jealousy in their relationships with other women. Some complain about them, grumbling: "Women can't be trusted" or "You can't count on women for support—they're so competitive!" Others hide or downplay their distress. Such pain and separation among women often goes undetected, but when unacknowledged and unresolved, it can keep them from supporting one another in hard times. Healing our relationships with other women requires us to practice compassion and maintain healthy boundaries.

Boundaries are often seen as barriers, shields that must be perpetually dragged around to use in self-defense against attacks. Subscribing to such a view can keep us in a state of agitation, chronically concerned about intercepting emotional blows and deflecting abusive behaviors. Instead, think of a boundary as a gate to your private garden, which you can open and close as desired. Closing the gate may feel uncomfortable at first, but remember that your need for protection is valid and does not have to be justified, defended, or explained. Start with easy boundaries and, as you get stronger, tackle more challenging ones. Healthy boundaries protect your well-being and inner harmony so you will be better equipped to help other women when called upon.

While setting a boundary, remember that you cannot control other people's reactions to it; you can only deliver the message with grace and love. If a boundary you set ends up hurting another woman's feelings, apologize if you can and recognize that women's relationships with other women improve when the individuals:

- Freely discuss each other's hardships
- Celebrate each other's breakthroughs and triumphs
- Actively nurture their friendship
- Remember that they are here to inspire and encourage women to shine as brightly as possible

Being Your Own Best Friend

One of the best ways to begin connecting with others is to pursue a more loving relationship with yourself, which will deepen your understanding and your compassion for other people's circumstances. For example, many women view their options for making friends as limited due to their beliefs about their appearance or competence. A woman I know sheepishly admitted she had gained forty pounds and was convinced that she couldn't make new friends because her wardrobe consisted of only sweat pants and T-shirts. My friend Sharron, a stay-at-home mom who recently divorced after twenty-five years of marriage, told me she'd been out of the socializing loop for so long that she felt inadequate and needed to know more or have better stories to share.

No matter what factors seem to be restricting your ability to make friends, pursuing a more loving relationship with yourself can help you see them not as obstacles but as limiting beliefs that can be overcome. You can begin creating a more loving relationship with yourself by recalling the words of people who have supported you in the past; writing affirmations to yourself; or recording and listening to self-affirming meditations associated with your personal strengths and dreams. As Diane von Fürstenberg said, "When a woman becomes her own best friend, life is easier."[3]

Taking Stock of Your Friendships

To form more supportive friendships with other women, it's important to periodically evaluate your current friendships to see which ones benefit your life. Consider whether your interests have recently changed and, if so, which friends help you feel seen and heard. A client recently told me she felt judged when her longtime girlfriends distanced themselves from her after she shared interest in exploring her sexual desires by trying new arousal techniques with her husband. Friends can also drift apart when one wants to expand her horizons, by traveling more or embarking on a journey of emotional or spiritual growth, while the other prefers to keep to familiar patterns.

To assess the staying power of your friendships, write your name, draw a circle around it, and along the perimeter write the names of the significant friends in your life. Moving around the circle one by one, draw an arrow toward your name from the names of friends whose support you receive and away from your name toward those of friends to whom you give support, in each instance letting the thickness of the arrow indicate the strength of the support. The friends with whom you share a reciprocal flow of support belong in your inner circle, and the others may not. Some may simply be casual acquaintances. Your connections with others may have become stagnant. Any time you notice a heavy feeling while thinking about certain people, consider whether you wish to continue investing time and energy in your relationship with them. If you find you're devoting yourself to women who don't support your best self, follow the advice of your inner Queen, who would say: "Go where you're celebrated, not where you're tolerated."

Tips for Selecting Your Angel Posse

After taking a good look at your current friendships, you may feel a call to connect with more women who are compatible and thus likely to become part of your angel posse. The following tips can help guide your search for friends with this potential.

Attracting an Angel Posse

Give yourself a reset. Travel to a place outside your normal environment, and open yourself to new possibilities, such as along the lush coast of Bali, beneath the Northern Lights in Iceland, or into a new neighborhood that has piqued your interest. At my annual retreat in Costa Rica, the participants leave the mundane world at home to connect with other "high-vibe" women, watching multicolored birds fly overhead while they splash in the waterfalls. At breakfast, they're introduced to a giant, bright green fruit, and they laugh themselves silly trying to pronounce its name, *guanabana*. Once, as a participant sank her teeth into the sweet white flesh, the juice dripping down her chin and hands, she exclaimed, "I feel like I'm taking a big bite of life!" The friendships born from this kind of shared experience—rooted in exploration, freedom, and pleasure—can foster some of the closest bonds and underscore how uplifting friendships can be.

Turn on your radar. You can find new friends almost anywhere as long as you tune in consciously to the "friend frequency." Kay was excited about landing her dream job as an advisor for women's education, but it meant leaving her longtime friends to move halfway around the world to Abu Dhabi. While settling into her new life in the Middle East, she adopted the habit of eavesdropping to determine whether she should introduce herself to people. Kay said, "I met Talia, my best friend in Abu Dhabi, that way. She was telling the hairdresser about her college-aged kids, which was a perfect opportunity to introduce myself. 'My college-aged daughters are coming for Christmas. What should we do?' I asked her. That led to Talia inviting me to go Christmas caroling in the desert that night." When you listen, you will find "your people," which often means people who are going through experiences and phases of life similar to your own. As you encounter others, it is useful to welcome positive people and avoid those who only notice problems in your situation.

Join a group or start one. Being part of a group of people with common interests is the easiest way to make friends. Explore groups in your area that offer activities you enjoy, such as cooking, photography, singing, yoga, gardening, birdwatching, hiking, painting, kayaking, journaling, dancing, or meditation. Online groups with live video classes are a convenient way to meet others and reach out to anyone with whom you resonate. Janet found her friendship group dwindling as she got older, so she decided to do something about it. When she met a woman she wanted to get to know, she invited her to the "unbook club" she had started. A small group of women Janet now considers good friends still gather at her house once a month for coffee or wine, and conversations that range from the heartache of having parents with dementia to the women's latest creative endeavors to new brands of lipstick. Sometimes they even talk about a book they're enjoying.

Volunteer for causes you believe in. Ask yourself what experiences in your life have made you want to reach out to others or contribute to society, then determine how and where you might use that passion to be of service. For example, Ginny discovered in her seventies that she had a passion for helping dogs, so she volunteered to foster and adopt some. Every day she went to a dog park with two fluffy foster dogs, Henry and his sister Honey. At first when told she should adopt their siblings, Ginny protested, "I'm too old to take on dogs. People my age shouldn't get puppies." However, when the pet adoption agency temporarily placed five mastiff puppies in her care and Ginny managed to care for them for six weeks without becoming stressed, she realized that her age hadn't diminished her abilities, and so she adopted the canine siblings. A bonus was that the human friendships she developed at the dog park became some of her most endearing.

Similarly, a friend who lost her sister to cancer now volunteers to sit with people during their chemotherapy infusions; and a massage therapist volunteers her services to several local nursing homes. The rich friendships that grow during such acts of generosity are often deeply rewarding.

Make friends with friends of friends. Befriending the friends of your friends can be a good way to expand your circle. When my friend Anne dragged me to her friend Gina's popular belly dance class, not only did I enjoy a fun way to keep my arms toned but also Gina and I became friends.

Once you have found a few new friends for your angel posse, make your relationships with them a high priority. In addition to getting together to socialize, don't hesitate to ask these individuals for help when you need it and to accept help when it's offered. No matter how strong and capable you are, remember that because you're human you need help.

Practice acceptance. Attracting and maintaining an angel posse can also be facilitated by practicing wholehearted acceptance of other women's strengths and weaknesses, as well as your own. A supportive, inspiring, and invaluable group of trusted girlfriends provides a lifeline unlike any other resource. This was made clear to me recently while spending a long weekend with three such friends. We gathered in a cozy cabin nestled in a pine forest, but we could have been just as happy in a tent because nothing fancy was required to support our friendship. We'd been friends for more than half our lives, accepting and nurturing one another through thick and thin. Being with these women reminded me of the hurdles I'd cleared, the lessons I'd learned, and who I really was. They'd been by my side through everything, lending steadiness, inspiration, and encouragement, and I'd been with them through the same.

As I looked around our small dinner table adorned with fresh flowers from the garden and saw my friends' faces glowing in candlelight, I realized that these women "got" me and I "got" them, with no need to prove anything. We never had to walk on eggshells with one another. We had no tally sheets or expectations of being paid back; in fact, each of us felt we had always gotten more in our interactions than we'd given. As I gazed deeply into each woman's eyes, my only thoughts were: "I completely accept you. I love everything about you."

The importance of having an angel posse—friends you can confide in and draw support from while navigating life—cannot be underestimated. They are the women:

- With whom you stay up late, sharing heart-to-heart talks
- Whom you love unconditionally, as they do you
- With whom you create timeless memories, act silly, and share jokes no one else understands
- Who support you when you feel lost, and vice versa
- Who inspire courage and wonder that enrich your life

When we lean on one another, learn from one another, and show up for one another no matter what we're going through, we cannot help but grow. It's an evolution that happens not just day by day but interaction by interaction, through little sparks of connection that build on one another and propel us forward, amplifying our joy.

BREATHING SPACE

Seen and unseen angels
show up for me when I need help.

I'm worthy of respect.

I enjoy giving and receiving with women of all ages.

PRACTICE

Becoming Your Own Best Friend

The longest, most important relationship you'll ever have is your relationship with yourself. But becoming a best friend to yourself takes practice. A simple way to begin is by doing one or more of these three exercises at least once a week:

- Sit quietly and recall one person who has encouraged you at some point in your life, perhaps a Wise Woman such as a teacher, grandmother, sister, aunt, or older friend. Remember how it felt when this person beamed love to you. Let your heart fill up with their love. Remember the feeling of being fully seen as they saw you, including your essence and the promise nestled within you.

- Write positive statements to yourself in a journal as if you were writing to a friend or relative. Be kind, generous, and forgiving as you express appreciation for all that you are.

- While drifting off to sleep at night, listen to a self-affirming meditation that expresses how you are inherently lovable, worthy of love, and endowed with valuable gifts and talents.

Attracting an Angel Posse

PRACTICE

Gathering Your Angel Posse

When preparing to gather your angel posse, call upon the nurturing strength of your Queen self as you follow this three-step strategy:

- Name three to five friends you spend the most time with, and ask yourself:

    Are they the mirrors I want in my life?
    Do they have the kinds of relationships that inspire me?
    Do I consider them successful at life?
    Do I feel as if they "get" me when I share my thoughts?
    What qualities do they bring out in me that I like?
    What qualities do they possess that I appreciate?
    Will they support my growth while honoring their own?

- Ask: Who in my life is out of alignment with who I currently am and who I aspire to be? Evaluate whether relationships that have changed over time continue to serve you. Then reduce the amount of time and energy you're investing in them and, if need be, grieve the loss.

- Ask: Who sees my greatness and helps me feel more alive? Reach out to these people and set up dates to spend time together. In cultivating closer relationships with them, you will know if they belong in your angel posse.

*Being your true self
despite fear, fatigue, doubt, and opposition...
will serve the world more than you can imagine.*

~Martha Beck

CHAPTER 9

Imagining a New Story of Aging

Crafting and Living Your Legacy

Imagining a new story of aging, one free of limiting beliefs, can dramatically change our expectations for later life and inspire us to expand the goals we hope to attain as part of our legacy. A growing body of research supports this shift to positive perceptions of aging. One study of social and emotional well-being in three hundred people ages eighteen to ninety-four was led by Laura Carstensen, psychology professor at Stanford University and author of *A Long Bright Future.* Her research showed that people over sixty-five are the most stable and optimistic of all adults, least likely to be anxious and depressed, most likely to have love in their lives, and able to live quite successfully on their own.[1] We can also draw inspiration from the experiences and words of wise elders—some famous, like the activist Gloria Steinem or the late author Maya Angelou, and others who are creating their legacy simply by living authentically and doing what makes them happy.

Philosopher and spiritual teacher Angeles Arrien, author of *The Second Half of Life,* informs us: "In many shamanic societies, if you came to a medicine person complaining of being disheartened, dispirited, or depressed, they would ask one of these four questions: When did you stop dancing? When did you stop singing? When did you stop being enchanted by stories? When did you stop finding comfort in the sweet territory of silence?"[2] When we ask ourselves these questions, the answers point to junctures where we may have abandoned our true selves as a result of subscribing to widespread myths about aging.

To assess women's limiting beliefs about growing older, I often ask them, "What frightens you most about aging?" Their usual responses are: "Running out of time" and "Losing people I love." The antidote for both fears is to build resilience by living a life as filled with appreciation, meaningful service, and fun as possible.

As Mary Pipher, author of *Women Rowing North*, says, "In our middle years and beyond we can have a sense that the runway is short."[3] We have a lot to explore, many talents to contribute, and don't want to look back in five or ten years wishing we had done certain things earlier. With the time we have left, we want to savor every experience and engage in activities that give our lives purpose and beauty.

Ultimately, only by envisioning what a satisfying, engaged life can look like are we able to build one. So whatever our age, it is time to start laying the groundwork for achieving this vision.

Living a Reality Worthy of Your Potential

Each woman has a unique gift the world needs. The goal is not to conform or shape yourself to meet society's expectations but to be gloriously yourself, reflective of your soul imprint. You are not here to fit in, keep the peace, or obey the rules but to be distinctive, extraordinary, and perhaps a bit strange—to add your piece to the great mosaic of humankind. In short, your mission is to craft a life that expresses your unique essence.

Imagining a New Story of Aging

You can do this by cultivating a readiness to engage and embrace your aliveness, as expressed by Joanna Macy and Chris Johnstone in their book *Active Hope*:

> Active hope is not wishful thinking.
> Active hope is not wishing to be rescued...
>   by some savior.
> Active hope is waking up to the beauty of life
>   on whose behalf we can act.
> We belong to this world.
> The web of life is calling us forth at this time.
> We've come a long way and are here to play our part.
> With active hope we realize that there are
>   adventures in store, strengths to discover,
>   and comrades to link arms with.
> Active hope is a readiness to discover the strengths
>   in ourselves and in others;
>   a readiness to discover the reasons for hope
>   and the occasions for love.
> A readiness to discover the size and strength of our hearts,
>   our quickness of mind, our steadiness of purpose,
>   our own authority, our love for life,
>   the liveliness of our curiosity,
>   the unsuspected well of deep patience and diligence,
>   the keenness of our senses and our
>   capacity to lead.
> None of these can be discovered in an armchair or
>   without risk.[4]

New Stories of Aging

A reliable catalyst for crafting new stories of aging is learning how other women facing its challenges have sustained their life forces, as recounted in the following two stories.

Janice Haynes's Story: Horses and Healing

When I interviewed Janice Haynes, she had just celebrated her seventy-second birthday. "I grew up on an island in New Hampshire as a nature-loving child," she told me. "My parents had a cabin on the lake. I had a rowboat when I was four, and I fished or walked around the island every day. I rode broom horses and exercised them daily in a circle in the grass." Her interaction with horses during childhood would later prove significant.

When Janice was ten years old, her family moved to Florida, where her love of nature was replaced by adherence to the dogmatic principles of a Baptist church, which formed her identity as a teenager. At nineteen, she began attending Wheaton College, at which point her beliefs collapsed, like falling dominos, and at age twenty-one she contemplated suicide. "I was searching for meaning and an identity, but I didn't have much to go on," she said. "I left college and hiked with a friend over the Rocky Mountains and down the other side of the Continental Divide. We found a guest ranch west of Denver, and the woman who ran the place fixed us breakfast and let me wash windows. She told me I could stay in one of the cabins if I helped with firewood. So I lived one cold winter in a little single-room cabin with an outhouse. I was heartsick, but reading great books of the Western world, which I'd found on a shelf in the cabin, helped me."

That winter Janice spent her days either by the woodstove reading or out snowshoeing with a dog she'd been allowed to borrow, surviving on $130 for food—rice, beans, and rabbits the neighbors had raised. "Every moment was so simple," she said. "I laughed when a weasel stole my last piece of bread and cheese. This Thoreau lifestyle suited me just fine." Still, Janice's will to live wasn't strong.

Eventually, she got lonesome and decided to hitchhike to Los Angeles to visit a friend. A burly trucker swung open his door, and she climbed into the front seat beside him. About fifty miles down the road when he showed her his pistol, it dawned on her that this could be a setup for an attack. "I didn't have much experience with men, and I wasn't sure what to do besides keep my eyes open," she said. "I willed myself to stay awake for twenty-four hours while he drove, talking nonstop. As the sky brightened the next morning, it occurred to me that staying awake to be sure she's safe is what a person would do if she wanted to live."

In her forties, Janice got married and had two baby girls. "I'm proudest of being a mom," she said. She homeschooled both girls, sold real estate for a living, and she and her husband traveled with the girls through Europe to show them more of the world.

After her daughters were grown, Janice had to rebuild her sense of self. While in her early sixties, she was diagnosed with malignant tumors in both breasts. She had a double lumpectomy at Memorial Sloan Kettering Cancer Center, but when the doctors wanted to follow up with chemo and radiation she declined since the radiation, aimed directly over her heart, was likely to affect her endurance and thus compromise her ability to hike, which she loved to do. Years later she was diagnosed with stage IV metastatic cancer and decided to pursue an alternative healing route. By that time, she had a horse and became a vegan after receiving from him the telepathic message: "Animals are not to be eaten." She also learned Reiki energy healing techniques and became a Reiki master.

With money that a dying aunt had left her, telling her to use it "for joy and life," Janice hiked in Scotland and traveled to the Findhorn community, where she learned to practice Qi Gong, took a class called Horse Sense and Soul, and met a Chinese woman who told her: "Follow the way of the horse—the passion of your heart—to get well."

This led Janice to study equine-facilitated psychotherapy through Eponaquest, which became key to her healing process. Later she attended a Psych-K class in Taos, New Mexico, with Dr. Bruce Lipton, the author of *The Biology of Belief.* Her tumors were stable, but Lipton told her emphatically, "They need to be gone. How long do you want to live?"

"I don't know—ten years?" she answered.

"Go for fifty years!" he exclaimed.

So Janice followed his advice and used Psych-K techniques to change her subconscious beliefs that were self-limiting and self-sabotaging. At her next scan, the tumors were gone, and she has remained tumor free.

Recently, she graduated from a course in healing touch for animals. "It's to help animals move through trauma and be happy from being fully seen. Horses see with their hearts, and now we're all learning to do this," Janice explained.

Janice continues to explore healing work, persistently going wherever it leads her. "When a door is presented, I don't wait for it to open. I open it and walk through," she stated. She's learning to become a therapeutic riding instructor for children with physical or emotional challenges. Her big dream, though, is to create a riding center. "I'd like to somehow be part of making the world better for horses," she said. "I still have a dream that I can change the lives of horses on this planet—love them, appreciate their great gifts, and give them decades full of kindness and generosity from humans."

When asked what advice she would give to younger women, she remarked: "We don't age except through programming in our brains. Aging isn't biological; it's learned behavior. I've noticed that my friends, even at forty, are already starting to 'get old.' But you can have years without aging. There's always a dream, a voice inside that wants to be heard. Trust that voice. Follow it. It will bless you and the people in your life."

Willie Lee Crews's Story: Sharecropping in the Deep South
At eighty-six, Willie Lee Crews was living independently in her own home in Birmingham, Alabama. She had grown up with her maternal grandparents on a plantation, where her family were sharecroppers. "It was hard work," she said, "but we had a house with windows one could close to shut out bad things, to shut out a world that we didn't want to infringe on us. We could allow people to see what we wanted them to see. We could love each other, play games, feel all the emotions of anger and joy, resentment and bitterness. We could laugh. We could run in the wind. We could roam through the woods with our two dogs and not allow the outside world to control us." By "outside world," Willie primarily meant the plantation owner and his riders, who spied on the sharecroppers to keep them in line. "We knew when to be quiet," Willie said.

On the plantation, Willie prayed for rain because when it rained the cotton would be too wet to pick and the children could go to school instead. Picking cotton in the fields meant Willie wasn't able to go to classes the full nine months of the school year; and there were no school buses for Black children until 1949, forcing them to get to town for school as best they could. Willie said she had excellent teachers, however. "They cared, and I remember all of them. We had a chemistry lab and a biology lab. I remember our music teacher. Every child had to take music."

She greatly admired her Grandmother Fannie. "She was this amazing woman who had a special kind of faith, and I knew early on that I wanted to be like her," Willie explained. "There were just things she knew—her care about people, her giving spirit. She could grow great vegetables, and she taught me to can and to quilt. Whatever she baked, she would share. She baked on ovens without controls, just wood and a fire. She could do seven-layer cakes and jelly cakes. She also made something my uncle called 'sad bread.' This was a mixture of whatever ingredients they had available, such as flour, butter, eggs, sugar, and milk. One day, when the plantation owner's riders came around, Fannie showed great courage. She sent her sons to hide among the trees, but one of them didn't make it in time. The riders claimed the boy was fifteen and therefore old enough to start working. Fannie stood up to them and protested: 'I carried this boy for nine months, so I ought to know how old he is. He ain't but ten, and he ain't going.'"

Willie still lives the beliefs she learned from her grandmother. "My grandmother did not believe in judging people. She believed in looking for good in them," she explains. She wants women today to realize that if someone wrongs us we don't have to carry those wrongs with us and worry about whether the person

Imagining a New Story of Aging

will experience consequences. "I don't have to stop living, waiting for someone to be punished," she notes. "Otherwise, I wouldn't be able to move forward. Taking up those wrongs puts a limit on how far I can go."

Willie also carries on her grandmother's belief in keeping a commitment. Fannie would tell Willie, "Granddaughter, if you see that man and he wants you and you want him, you marry that man. If he does not do what he's supposed to do, you still keep your commitment. But if the day should come when you have to leave, you walk clean. Walk out that door, and you close it and you don't look back."

As part of her legacy, Willie plans to write stories about her family. "I often feel that my mind is running down home, especially when experiences from childhood come flooding in," she says. She is also collecting memorabilia, including books about Black children, to help others better understand the past experiences of Blacks in the South. "Growing up, we had the Bible, and if we found a magazine I'd read the stories and then plaster our walls with them for insulation from the cold wind," she explains. Additionally, Willie is shaping her legacy by enlisting support to provide sports programs for the young people in her childhood community, one of the poorest in the country. She's currently working with the staff at her former high school to repair the gym, a project for which she has helped raise over $500,000.

Willie believes she will leave behind a legacy of knowledge about what she has witnessed, stating, "I've been in situations where implications have been made about Black children or Black people in general, and I can't listen to that and not say something. I hope I pass along to my children and grandchildren the idea that when you speak, know what you're talking about. Have some evidence and facts. My charge was to teach and be an example, to try to live the best example I could." Willie feels an important aspect of her legacy is reflecting how love helps us rise above daily struggles, "knowing the richness of love, knowing that I'm loved no matter the issues, no matter the struggles—and that includes more than just the love from my family."

It is evident from this story that Willie, like Janice, has learned something unexpected about the wisdom years—that this is a fertile time when we can use every insight and breakthrough that comes our way to compose a new story of aging in which we embrace life with curiosity, gratitude, and a willingness to be of service. Each leap we make signals a profound inner awakening—a time of rebirth, when we know the part we play in the symphony of life.

Living Large

Living large means living according to our true nature to reach our highest potential, which may occur only later in life. Oak trees don't start producing acorns until they are about fifty years old, at which point they can generate over fifty thousand acorns each year. Among killer whales, or orcas, it is postmenopausal females that are perhaps most vital to their survival. These grandmother whales pass along information on the best hunting grounds to the children and grandchildren. In times of food scarcity, when the salmon supply is low, it is the oldest post-reproductive females who lead their pods. If the grandmothers die, the group doesn't do nearly as well.[5] Comparable to oak trees and orcas, we humans build up energy over the years so that later in life we can share our abundant gifts with the world.

Imagining a New Story of Aging

We gather such energy by having the courage to live with an open heart, holding nothing back, owning and transcending our fears. An indigenous elder, living large in her nineties, shared with me this simple guidance for a happy life: "In each day that is born we experience the miracle of life. Let's receive each dawn with gratitude for the path that opens before us. Let's thank each dusk for the learning on our path, the renewal that will come in the night. Let's thank the universe for all that we are and for each day that allows us to be reborn."

A life lived large does not necessarily mean a famous life. Think of an elder you admire not so much for her deeds as for her radiance, the glow of her character, and her patience, courage, and tireless optimism. In aspiring to such a life, listen to your inner allies. Perhaps your Queen self is inviting you to "slow down and simply be." Or maybe your Maiden self is nudging you to pursue a long-buried dream, such as writing a memoir or making art with a child. Then, heart first, go play your unique part in the web of life, which will soon have you lighting up others in your midst.

Ultimately, the greatest legacies we leave in this world are the lives we touch, the people we inspire to open up to more of their own potential. So it is that our highest purpose and most treasured offering is to be radiant for no reason other than simply being alive.

BREATHING SPACE

I'm ready to discover and celebrate my many strengths.

I am a strong and boldly colored thread
in this beautiful sacred tapestry.

It's time for me to share my greatness with the world.

PRACTICE

What Do You Stand For and Who Stands with You?

I was introduced to the following standing meditation by Gail Larsen, author of the book *Transformational Speaking*, during a retreat for visionary leaders outside Santa Fe, New Mexico. Gail instructed us to walk into the desert and, following our intuitive guidance, choose a large wooden stick to represent our seen and unseen guides—the supportive people in our lives today and our ancestors. She then asked us to connect to our rage, acknowledging what we will no longer stand for.

As the sun set, we sat in silence on the wide stone patio, decorating our staffs with yarn, beads, and feathers. Each person then stood and voiced the allegiances she felt in her heart, such as: "I stand for the children. I stand for the animals of the earth. I stand for the trees. I stand for the oceans. I stand for women who are forced to be silent."

To do this practice yourself:

- Find a stick and decorate it as you wish, with materials meaningful to you.
- Fasten one feather to the top, pointing upward.
- Sense the aliveness in your staff.
- Say from your heart what you stand for.
- Feel yourself supported by your ancestors and the people currently in your life who help you.
- Stand with your staff five minutes or longer each day to strengthen your commitment.

*We begin to find and become ourselves
when we notice how we are already found,
already truly, entirely, wildly, messily, marvelously
who we were born to be.*

~Anne Lamott

CHAPTER 10

Awakening to Your Divine Blueprint

Realizing Your Radiance

There is a vast intelligence for each of us to tap in to when we understand where we came from and the inner resources that connect us to our origins. That intelligence, often referred to as our divine blueprint, contains our countless life experiences and leads us to the discovery of our life purpose, the unique "assignments" we each agreed to carry out in this lifetime.

The presence of a divine blueprint was reinforced within me a few years ago when, while deep in meditation, I saw a vision of a place that felt familiar from the distant past—an island far across the ocean, lush with tangled green vines and brightly colored flowers, and imbued with warm air and a peaceful atmosphere, where I lived among women and men who communicated telepathically with one another. On the shores of this island were giant black rocks with clear quartz crystals inside. People who were ill arrived in boats and were carried to sit or lie near the rocks. I was one of many healers who directed energy from the crystals to anyone needing to be restored to wellness. After enjoying this scene for a while, I looked out at the horizon and saw three pillars of light moving toward me. With tears streaming down my face, I cried out, "The women are coming!" As these pillars of light drew closer and brighter, I thought they represented women from around the world who would be joining me to usher in a new age of empowerment for women.

Women from around the world have in fact been connecting with me. And I now realize that those three pillars of light represented the Maiden, the Queen, and the Wise Woman—the archetypal allies who continually support us as we progress in fulfilling our potential. These three energies have guided us on our journeys as we've broken free from the fear and pain of the past, turned our attention to our bodies' wisdom, and trusted our intuitive urgings. They have helped us remember our divine essence. As we continue our journeys of transformation, these three allies, along with our ancestors, stand ready to assist us.

Awakening to our divine blueprint is vital for not only uncovering our life plan but also renewing our inner being for our own benefit and that of others. It is time for women to embrace such knowledge and trust their wisdom so they can play the vital roles that are needed on the planet.

We need to embrace the bull's message that our essence "cannot be contained." Our tasks at this point are to follow our intuitive impulses and risk being called crazy; to choose the more joyful, self-fulfilling path, where we no longer feel frustrated or stuck; and to walk forward along this path of greatest potential, prepared to ask for the support we need along the way from our guides, friends, and family.

Awakening of the Feminine Cocreator

Currently, in a world gripped by the coronavirus pandemic, with the World Health Organization reporting millions of confirmed cases of Covid-19 globally and several million related deaths,[1] many people feel confused, unbalanced, or lost. Some say this is the great change of the age predicted centuries ago by Nostradamus, the Aztecs, the Hopi, the Maya, and many other ancient traditions.[2] And while a virus sparked this worldwide crisis, an underlying pandemic of racial and economic inequality fuels the fire. Now people around the world are being presented with an opportunity to shift to modes of connection and cocreation as never before, to focus not only on personal needs but also on the higher good of humanity and all life on earth.

As a collective, we have a choice between trying to go back to the way things were or taking a new road. Do we settle for the old story of separation and hide in fear, or do we awaken to the truth that we're all interconnected and our unified commitment has the potential to create a new reality? Resilience is the basis of all life on earth. This doesn't mean everything will bounce back to where it was but that surviving a process of challenge and change is part of what it means to be human. Because our ancestors have survived famines, genocide, and cataclysmic change, the knowledge of how to survive harsh times is encoded in our DNA.

As old paradigms crumble, we sense the awakening of collective feminine energy that the late Barbara Marx Hubbard, founder of the Foundation for Conscious Evolution, called the "feminine cocreator." The rise of this feminine energy is essential to the survival of humanity and the regeneration of planet Earth. If we believe that each of us comes to the planet for a purpose, then being here at this time in history offers us the opportunity to be part of a collective quantum leap forward. The task remains for each of us to ask ourselves two crucial questions: What part am I being called to play? What is mine to *be* and *do*? Together, with courage and renewed clarity, we can help manifest the vision of a more just and healthy world for ourselves, our loved ones, and humanity.

Using Your Gifts to Make a Difference

While growing up, many of us were taught to stay in our place and accept the status quo. Even those who could see the brokenness in the world around us were told there was nothing we could do about it; that's just the way things were. But what if our inner longings and dreams are more growth promoting than the circumstances we see? What if the dreams we hold inside are meant to be unleashed? If we don't imagine change and act on our visions despite doubters who challenge us, we'll get what we've always gotten. As expressed in the Apple computer ad from the late 1990s that flashed images of iconic visionaries, such as Martha Graham, Martin Luther King Jr., and Amelia Earhart, then ended with the message "It's the ones we call crazy who change the world," the people who courageously take action to fulfill their longings and achieve their dreams are the ones who create the flourishing of changes crucial to humanity.

While listening to women over the past twenty years, I've heard their longings and found them inspiring. Women want to take a deep breath and rest. Women want all children to have a safe home and enough to eat. Women want to see more kindness and less suffering.

Imagine what our world would look like if there were a rebirth of reverence for women in all stages of life. Then if women, trusting themselves and in conscious alliance with others, used their gifts to make a difference, miraculous things would happen. Relationships would be healed. Corruption would be replaced by justice and equality. New regenerative systems for food, education, health, and energy production would prevail. Children would inspire us to see the world as a friendly place. The water and air would be clean, and the animals and plants would thrive. Menopausal and postmenopausal women in all cultures would become role models, mentors, and wisdom carriers for the younger generations, revered by a society that respects the experience and insight of sage elders.

Fortunately, increasing numbers of women are now gaining awareness of their influence and are coming together to create change in the world. In their communities, young women are finding their voices and demanding justice for the earth and her people. These courageous activists need us, the Wise Women, to affirm their truth-telling and collaboration and to ground them in the certainty that change is possible and heart-to-heart resonance is already occurring globally, altering outdated structures and roles. Each of us has a vital part to play in this time when nothing seems normal yet we feel our hopes and dreams swelling inside us.

As we revive and celebrate the feminine archetypes of the Maiden, Queen, and Wise Woman, we create circles of reciprocity where women of all ages can enjoy a flow of giving and receiving strength and support and can see women's cycles as a vital expression of the inner wild power that is our birthright. Nurtured in these circles of sisterhood, we regain our ability to listen to our intuition, value our female nature, and dream into reality the more beautiful and just world we imagine. We reclaim our heritage, challenging the status quo and changing obsolete paradigms, illusions historically passed off as truths. Picking up these long-forgotten threads, we weave them into a rich tapestry that sustains everyone everywhere. So it is that living our wisdom supports all life on the planet.

By shining our light into the world, we give permission for people in darkness to shine their light. In allowing ourselves to radiate the frequency of pure love as we step out to serve, we create a ripple in the energy grid around the planet—a strong current that vibrates in remembrance of our divine blueprint, sparking us to live our greatness. We stand at the forefront, living a new story of conscious aging for ourselves, our world, and future generations.

BREATHING SPACE

The gifts I share make a positive difference.

I believe in my audacious dreams.

I trust my knowing.

PRACTICE

Claiming Your "I Am" Presence

To fully embody your power, it is essential to uncover and proclaim who you truly are, as described in this practice. To begin, single out one of your greatest dreams and imagine yourself having achieved it. Then ask yourself, "How would I need to be to really achieve this dream?" List the necessary qualities, writing "I am" before each one, as indicated below. Because thoughts create reality, the qualities you list will be those that emerge, so be sure to record only those you most value, such as: "I am strong (resilient, worthy, connected, safe, honest, loved, patient, forgiving, creative, supported)."

Qualities:
(I am) _____
(I am) _____
(I am) _____

Since your list of statements will support you in achieving not only that dream but many more, review your list carefully to be certain the values it reflects are those you envision as enduring.

When you are happy with your statements, stand up and read each one aloud. To amplify its power, press together the tip of your index finger and the tip of your thumb, thereby anchoring the statement. Proclaiming these carefully chosen attributes rewires your brain circuits to reinforce thoughts that serve you rather than defeat you. Feel your body adjust to make room for this new way of being. Feel your spine lengthen as, looking outward, you see your dream manifested.

PRACTICE

Connecting to Your Wise Woman Self

To assess the progress you have made in awakening to your divine blueprint, periodically reconnect with your Wise Woman self. To gain her perspective, imagine that you are in a meadow on a clear, sunlit day, filled with joy as you stroll along, surrounded by wildflowers and butterflies, your hair caressed by the breeze. At the edge of the meadow, you see a dirt path covered in soft green moss and, guided by birdsong, follow it through a forest infused with scents of balsam, fir, and cedar until you see a small house nestled in a clearing. You step onto the porch, knock softly on the door, and hear a woman's voice say, "Please come in." You open the door and cross the threshold.

To your right, you see a simple yet inviting room with two cozy chairs and a small table set with a teapot and two cups. In one of the chairs is an enchanting older woman who smiles warmly and invites you to sit in the other chair. You settle into the chair, which seems to fit you perfectly, and you relax as she gazes into your eyes. You study her face and ask her name; she responds quietly. She pours you a cup of spicy orange tea and tells you, with a twinkle in her eye, how curious she is about your life's journey and how it is evolving. She then asks you the following questions, and the answers seem to cascade from you effortlessly:

- Are you being kinder to yourself?
- Are you finding you can trust your intuition more?
- Do you feel less alone? Are friends showing up in your life?

- Are you doing less striving and more savoring?
- What is your body teaching you as you listen to it?
- What are some of the positive changes you're celebrating?
- In this second spring of your life, what are you looking forward to?

The woman listens intently, nodding now and then, until you've fully expressed your thoughts. Then, with a knowing smile, she encourages you to take the next steps on your journey into the empowered, sensually fulfilled, joyful life that awaits you.

You feel your body vibrate with the energy of love as you hear her words: "Radiant Sister, remember to befriend your three allies—the Maiden, Queen, and Wise Woman. Indulge in goblets of endorphins, and let pleasure have her way with you. Forgive yourself and others. Gather your angel posse, and go where you're celebrated. Honor your body. Trust your voice. Stand in the power of your truth. You matter. Your voice matters. Your life matters. You came here to create amazing things. Thank you for shining your light. The world needs you, wise and awake. So go now and live your greatness from your brilliance, courage, and magic."

After one last sip of tea, you stand up as your Wise Woman rises from her chair to give you a hug. She whispers in your ear that you can come back any time for her help. You bow in gratitude and prepare to leave. You open the front door and, breathing in the forest fragrance, walk back down the mossy path into the meadow. With each step you take, you feel more curious and excited about living your wild orgasmic wisdom.

RESOURCES

Following are recommended books, websites, and mobile apps for informed decision-making on issues related to menopause, perimenopause, sexual health, nutrition, mental and emotional health, and spiritual growth.

Menopause

The Alchemy of Menopause: The Journey of Stepping into Our Power and Becoming Who We Truly Are by Cathy Skipper. Offers a framework based on C. G. Jung's concepts of inner alchemy, along with suggested essential oils, to help women understand how the physical experiences of menopause are the body's way of triggering profound transformation.

The Estrogen Question: Know Before You Say "No" to HRT by Sandra Rice, MD. A comprehensive look at hormone replacement therapy, with up-to-date information about its benefits and risks.

The Menopause Switch: Disrupt Aging and Live Your Best Life Past Midlife by Dr. Carissa Alinat. Offers science-based, effective, and natural solutions for hot flashes, weight gain, insomnia, and the end of intimacy.

The Secret Life of Hormones: Finding Hormone Balance for a Better Life by Dr. Zoe Zawalick. Clarifies the confusing changes of perimenopause, helping readers bring their hormones into balance, maintain their weight, and feel good again.

Wild Power: Discover the Magic of Your Menstrual Cycle and Awaken the Feminine Path to Power by Alexandra Pope and Sjanie Hugo Wurlitzer. Provides information to assist readers in working with their inner seasons to pace their energy, calm their nervous systems, and gain insight into their overall well-being.

The Wisdom of Menopause: Creating Physical and Emotional Health and Healing, (5th ed.) by Christiane Northrup, MD. A groundbreaking book that presents a new vision of midlife as not simply a collection of physical symptoms to be fixed but rather a mind-body revolution that brings the greatest opportunity for growth since adolescence.

Yoga for Osteoporosis: The Complete Guide by Loren Fishman, MD, and Ellen Saltonstall, MD. A comprehensive guide that helps readers understand osteoporosis and offers a spectrum of exercises for beginners and experts, including classical yoga poses, as well as physiologically sound adapted poses, with easy-to-follow instructions and photographs.

www.health.harvard.edu/topics/menopause—Articles and up-to-date research on women's unique health concerns, including perimenopause, menopause, bioidentical hormones, and mental health.

www.menopause.org—Website of the North American Menopause Society (NAMS), designed to help readers find providers who have passed an exam demonstrating their knowledge of menopause.

MenoPro—Free mobile app from the North American Menopause Society that helps patients and clinicians work together to personalize treatment decisions on the basis of preferences (hormone vs. non-hormone options), taking into account medical history and risk factors.

Resources

www.project-aware.org—Website of the Association of Women for the Advancement of Research and Education, offering objective and comprehensive health information related to perimenopause, menopause, and postmenopause.

www.redschool.net—Website featuring menstrual knowledge, provided by the authors of *Wild Power* to enhance the understanding of menopause and postmenopause.

www.womenshealth.gov/menopause—Website of the National Women's Health Information Center, designed to address frequently asked questions about menopause, including symptoms, treatments, and sexual health.

Perimenopause
The Mayo Clinic Menopause Solution: A Doctor's Guide to Relieving Hot Flashes, Enjoying Better Sex, Sleeping Well, Controlling Your Weight, and Being Happy! by Stephanie S. Faubion, MD, NCMP. Offers information for women about taking charge of their own health and getting the best care from their doctors, including material on perimenopause, premature menopause, menopause symptoms, and a wide variety of therapies to enhance health.

www.acog.org/womens-health—Website of the American College of Obstetricians and Gynecologists, featuring a searchable database on perimenopause, menopause, and sexual health.

Sexual Health
Come as You Are: The Surprising New Science That Will Transform Your Sex Life by Emily Nagoski, PhD. Presents

research indicating that the most important factor for women in creating and sustaining a fulfilling sex life is not what occurs in bed but how they feel about it and that stress, mood, trust, and body image are not peripheral factors in women's sexual well-being but central to it.

Living an Orgasmic Life: Heal Yourself and Awaken Your Pleasure by Xanet Pailet. For women who find sex challenging and are alienated from their erotic nature due to sexual abuse, trauma, or inability to surrender to pleasure, sustain intimacy, or feel sexually empowered.

Mating in Captivity: Unlocking Erotic Intelligence by Esther Perel. Offers a new take on intimacy and sex, and demonstrates how more exciting, playful sex is possible in long-term relationships.

Sex for One: The Joy of Selfloving by Betty Dodson, PhD. The classic guide to fully enjoying the pleasures of self-love; full of warmth, intelligence, and informative line drawings by a renowned sex educator.

Tantra: Sex for the Soul—Easy Steps to More Intimacy, Passion, Pleasure & Love by Niyaso Carter. An audiobook, CD, or Spotify guide to tantra and a vibrant sex life that is entertaining, lighthearted, and instructional, taking into account men's and women's differing needs for support, and presenting exercises and practices that are easy to follow and fun to do.

www.goodvibes.com—A safe and nonjudgmental educational environment that promotes sexual pleasure and empowerment, and offers online shopping for high-quality sex toys and books, with discreet shipping options.

Resources

www.omgyes.com—Practical techniques to enhance pleasure, solo or as a couple; the distilled wisdom of twenty thousand women ages eighteen to ninety-five presented in short, honest videos.

www.sexualityresources.com—A sex education resource center operated by two women—a physician and a sex counselor—offering information for people of all ages, orientations, and body types, as well as products for sex before and after menopause, based on current sex science.

Nutrition

Healthy Aging: A Lifelong Guide to Your Well-Being by Andrew Weil, MD. A book about longevity that separates myth from fact about life extension; discusses herbs, hormones, and anti-aging "medicines"; and provides an anti-inflammatory eating plan that protects the immune system, as well as exercise, breathing, and stress-management techniques to benefit mind and body.

Medical Medium Life-Changing Foods: Save Yourself and the Ones You Love with the Hidden Healing Powers of Fruits & Vegetables by Anthony William. Information about the capacity of over fifty foods to relieve hypertension, brain fog, thyroid imbalances, migraines, and other conditions.

The Menopause Diet Plan: A Natural Guide to Managing Hormones, Health, and Happiness by Hillary Wright, MEd, RDN, and Elizabeth M. Ward, MS, RD. A plant-based eating plan that encourages a positive, fad-free approach to managing physical and emotional health during perimenopause and menopause.

The Menopause Reset: Get Rid of Your Symptoms and Feel Like Your Younger Self Again by Dr. Mindy Pelz. Information that helps women reset their nutrition, weight, and health during their menopausal years.

The Plant Power Doctor: A Simple Prescription for a Healthier You by Dr. Gemma Newman. Recipes, articles, and podcast interviews on plant-powered eating to transform health.

www.galvestondiet.com. An anti-inflammatory approach to nutrition developed by Mary Claire Haver, MD, to help women in menopause lose weight, have more energy, and create sustainable, healthy habits.

Mental and Emotional Health
Daring Greatly: How the Courage to Be Vulnerable Transforms the Way We Live, Love, Parent, and Lead by Brené Brown, PhD, LMSW. A book dispelling the cultural myth that vulnerability is weakness and offering a practice and new vision fostering the benefits of vulnerability.

The Desire Map: A Guide to Creating Goals with Soul by Danielle LaPorte. A dream-fulfilling system for actualizing the innermost desire to feel good.

Healing Your Aloneness: Finding Love and Wholeness through Your Inner Child by Erika J. Chopich and Margaret Paul. Discusses how people can reconnect with their inner child to short-circuit self-destructive patterns, resolve fears and conflicts, and build satisfying relationships.

From Heartbreak to Wholeness: The Hero's Journey to Joy by Kristine Carlson. A moving story about the sudden death of the author's spouse, revealing a process of healing that goes beyond ordinary prescriptions for getting through hard times and offers a map for navigating the journey from loss to love, hope, and vision.

Loving What Is: Four Questions That Can Change Your Life by Byron Katie and Stephen Mitchell. A self-inquiry approach that enhances the ability to see personal difficulties in a different light and demonstrates, through clear examples, how to use the method.

There Is Nothing Wrong with You: Going Beyond Self-Hate by Cheri Huber. A book that explains the origin of self-hate, how self-hate works, how to identify it, and how to go beyond it.

Transformational Speaking: If You Want to Change the World, Tell a Better Story by Gail Larsen. A proven program that liberates the "speaker within" and transforms even the reluctant orator into an agent of change.

Untamed by Glennon Doyle. A poignant memoir in which the "patron saint of female empowerment" explores the joy and peace to be discovered when people stop striving to meet others' expectations and begin to trust themselves enough to set boundaries, make peace with their bodies, honor their anger and heartbreaks, and unleash their truest instincts.

Women Rowing North: Navigating Life's Currents and Flourishing as We Age by Mary Pipher. A *New York Times* bestseller guide to wisdom, authenticity, and bliss for women as they age.

Spiritual Growth

Active Hope: How to Face the Mess We're in without Going Crazy by Joanna Macy and Chris Johnstone. A resource for discovering new strengths and a wider network of allies to more fully contribute to a society that supports the flourishing of life.

The Four Spiritual Laws of Prosperity: A Simple Guide to Unlimited Abundance by Edwene Gaines. An empowering exploration of the true meaning of prosperity in the effort to achieve a life of spiritual and material abundance.

Mary Magdalene Revealed: The First Apostle, Her Feminist Gospel & the Christianity We Haven't Tried Yet by Meggan Watterson. A Harvard-trained theologian's verse-by-verse illumination of Mary's gospel, revealing a radical love at the heart of the Christian story and a pronouncement that people are not sinful and should not feel ashamed or unworthy for being human.

The Second Half of Life: Opening the Eight Gates of Wisdom by Angeles Arrien. A guide to spiritual maturity—deepening valuable relationships, reclaiming creative talents, and shifting focus from ambition to meaning—for those seeking to become exceptional elders.

Women Who Run with the Wolves: Myths and Stories of the Wild Woman Archetype by Clarissa Pinkola Estés, PhD. A combination of time-honored stories and contemporary casework demonstrating that the "wild woman" is innately healthy, passionate, and wise, and giving readers a new sense of self-confidence and purpose.

NOTES

Introduction
1. Maoshing Ni, *Second Spring: Dr. Mao's Hundreds of Natural Secrets for Women to Revitalize and Regenerate at Any Age* (New York: Atria, 2009), 6.
2. Ni, *Second Spring*, 9.
3. I interviewed a diverse group of over one hundred women, ages thirty-eight to eighty-five, via phone, email, and in person.
4. Mark Cartwright, "The Pillow Book," *World History Encyclopedia*, updated April 20, 2017, https://www.ancient.eu/the_pillow_book.

Chapter 1
1. Kathy Weiser, "The Cherokee Trail of Tears," *Legends of America*, updated May 2020, https://www.legendsofamerica.com/na-trailtears.
2. A story told by Edwene Gaines at a women's retreat, Rock Ridge Retreat Center, Valley Head, Alabama, March 2016.
3. Clarissa Pinkola Estés, *Women Who Run with the Wolves: Myths and Stories of the Wild Woman Archetype* (New York: Ballantine Books, 1996), 200.

Chapter 2
1. "Menopause 101: A Primer for the Perimenopausal," North American Menopause Society, accessed January 21, 2020, http://www.menopause.org/for-women/menopauseflashes/menopause-symptoms-and-treatments/menopause-101-a-primer-for-the-perimenopausal.
2. Adriana Velez, "Menopause Is Different for Women of Color," Endocrine Web, updated May 18, 2020, https://www.endocrineweb.com/menopause-different-women-color.
3. Velez, "Menopause Is Different."
4. "Essential Oils for Sleep," American Sleep Association, accessed August 17, 2020, https://www.sleepassociation.org/sleep-treatments/essential-oils-for-sleep.

5. "Adrenal Fatigue Diet," Women's Health Network, December 22, 2020, https://www.womenshealthnetwork.com/adrenal-fatigue-and-stress/the-adrenal-fatigue-diet.

6. Zach Bush, "Nutrition: The Gut Brain Axis and Human Performance," December 3, 2020, in *Global Health Education Podcast*, podcast, website, 1:38:58, https://zachbushmd.com/knowledge-nutrition/?mc_cid=edc56b31f1&mc_eid=68006fb264.

7. Mindy Pelz, *The Menopause Reset: Get Rid of Your Symptoms and Feel Like Your Younger Self Again* (Las Vegas, NV: Lifestyle Entrepreneurs Press, 2020), 47.

8. Pelz, *Menopause Reset*, 48.

9. Hrefna Palsdottir, "Nine Benefits of Maca Root and Potential Side Effects," *Healthline*, updated October 30, 2016, https://www.healthline.com/nutrition/benefits-of-maca-root.

10. Anne Loehr, "How Menopause Silently Affects 27 Million Women at Work Every Day," Fast Company, updated February 17, 2016, https://www.fastcompany.com/3056703/how-menopause-silently-affects-27-million-women-at-work-every-day.

11. Ni, *Second Spring*, 320.

12. "The Witch Trials," *Western Civilization* (course content for Lumen Learning), accessed November 2, 2019, https://courses.lumenlearning.com/suny-hccc-worldhistory/chapter/the-witch-trials.

13. Christiane Northrup, *The Wisdom of Menopause: Creating Physical and Emotional Health and Healing*, 5th ed. (New York: Bantam, 2020), 52.

14. Clarissa Pinkola Estés, *The Late Bloomer: Myths & Stories of the Wise Woman Archetype*, read by the author (Louisville, CO: Sounds True, 2012), audiobook, 7:50:00.

Chapter 3

1. Dolly Parton, "PMS Blues," September 27, 1994, Columbia, track number 23 on *Heartsongs: Live from Home*, LP vinyl.

2. Gillian Anderson and Jennifer Nadel, "The Truth Is Out There (About Menopause)," *Lenny Letter*, March 7, 2017, https://www.lennyletter.com/story/the-truth-is-out-there-about-menopause.

Notes

3. "Exploring Deborah Tannen's Sex, Lies, and Conversation," PhD diss., updated January 26, 2021, https://phdessay.com/exploring-deborah-tannens-sex-lies-and-conversation.
4. Rob Pascale and Lou Primavera, "Male and Female Brains," *Psychology Today* (April 25, 2019), https://www.psychologytoday.com/us/blog/so-happy-together/201904/male-and-female-brains.

Chapter 4
1. Aubrey Marcus, "Ecstasy in Life and Death with Dr. Zach Bush, MD," December 2, 2020, in *Aubrey Marcus Podcast #285*, podcast, website, 1:57:00, https://www.aubreymarcus.com/blogs/aubrey-marcus-podcast/ecstasy-in-life-and-death-with-dr-zach-bush-md-amp-285.

Chapter 5
1. Pema Chödrön, *When Things Fall Apart: Heart Advice for Difficult Times* (Boulder, CO: Shambhala Publications, 1997), 14.
2. Matt Kahn, "The Pain of Loss," *All for Love*, YouTube video, 1:33:18, June 12, 2018, https://www.youtube.com/watch?v=0kXVcGGwqwA.
3. Kahlil Gibran, *Kahlil Gibran: The Collected Works* (New York: Alfred A. Knopf, 2007), 568.
4. Etty Hillesum, *An Interrupted Life and Letters from Westerbork* (New York: Henry Holt, 1996), 93.

Chapter 6
1. Loren Eiseley, *The Unexpected Universe* (New York: Harcourt Brace & Company, 1972), 24.
2. William T. Hornaday, *The Extermination of the American Bison 1886–87* (Washington, DC: Government Printing Office, 1889).
3. Anne M. R. Agur and Arthur F. Dalley, *Grant's Atlas of Anatomy*, 13th ed. (Baltimore, MD: Lippincott Williams & Wilkins, 2013), 804.
4. Agur and Dalley, *Grant's Atlas of Anatomy*, 198.

Notes

5. Azra Bertrand and Seren Bertrand, *Womb Awakening: Initiatory Wisdom from the Creatrix of All Life* (Rochester, VT: Bear & Company, 2017), 161.

6. Joanna Macy and Sam Mowe, "The Work That Reconnects," *Tricycle* (Spring 2015), https://tricycle.org/magazine/work-reconnects.

7. Joanna Macy and Molly Young Brown, *Coming Back to Life: The Updated Guide to the Work That Reconnects* (Gabriola Island, BC: New Society Publishers, 2014), 6–14.

Chapter 7

1. Esther Perel. *Mating in Captivity: Unlocking Erotic Intelligence* (New York: Harper Paperbacks, 2017), 202.

2. William Acton, *The Functions and Disorders of the Reproductive Organs in Childhood, Youth, Adult Age, and Advanced Life: Considered in Their Physiological, Social, and Moral Relations*, 3rd ed. (London: Churchill, 1862), 101.

3. Eve Ensler, *The Vagina Monologues* (New York: Villard Books, 2001), 51.

4. Regina Nuzzo, "The Science of Orgasm," *Los Angeles Times*, September 15, 2014, https://www.latimes.com/health/la-he-orgasm11feb11-story.html.

5. Debby Herbenick et al., "Women's Experiences with Genital Touching, Sexual Pleasure, and Orgasm: Results from a U.S. Probability Sample of Women Ages 18 to 94," *Journal of Sex and Marital Therapy* 44 (2018): 204, https://doi.org/10.1080/0092623X.2017.1346530.

6. Zawn Villines, "What to Know about Vaginal Lubrication," *Medical News Today*, September 25, 2019, https://www.medicalnewstoday.com/articles/326450.

7. Herbenick, "Women's Experiences."

8. David-Michel Davies, "Rob Perkins and Lydia Daniller, Founders of OMGYes," December 12, 2017, in *The Webby Podcast* S2 EP8, podcast, website, 0:34:00, https://play.acast.com/s/webbypodcast/s2ep8-robperkinsandlydiadaniller-foundersofomgyes.

9. Niyaso Carter, *Tantra: Sex for the Soul—Easy Steps to More Intimacy, Passion, Pleasure & Love* (Paia, HI: Sacred Loving Institute, 2016), audiobook read by the author, 6:13:00.
10. Richard Miller, *The Magical and Ritual Use of Perfumes* (Rochester, VT: Inner Traditions, 1990), 65.

Chapter 8
1. Julianne Holt-Lunstad et al., "Loneliness and Social Isolation as Risk Factors for Mortality," *Perspectives on Psychological Science* 10, no. 2 (2015): 230, https://doi.org/10.1177/1745691614568352.
2. S. E. Taylor et al., "Biobehavioral Responses to Stress in Females: Tend-and-Befriend, Not Fight-or-Flight," *Psychological Review* 107, no. 3 (2000): 419, https://doi.org/10.1037/0033-295X.107.3.411.
3. Diane von Fürstenberg, *The Woman I Wanted to Be* (New York: Simon & Schuster, 2014), 128.

Chapter 9
1. Laura Carstensen, *A Long Bright Future: An Action Plan for a Lifetime of Happiness, Health, and Financial Security* (New York: Public Affairs, 2011), 16.
2. Angeles Arrien, Foreword to *Maps to Ecstasy: The Healing Power of Movement* by Gabrielle Roth (Novato, CA: New World Library, 1998), xv-xvi.
3. Terry Gross and Mary Pipher, "Aging Offers Women Enormous Possibilities for Growth," February 27, 2019, in *Fresh Air*, produced by WHYY, podcast, MP3 audio, 0:19:55, http://www.npr.org/2019/02/27/698535498/aging-offers-women-enormous-possibilities-for-growth-says-author.
4. Joanna Macy and Chris Johnstone, *Active Hope: How to Face the Mess We're in without Going Crazy* (Novato, CA: New World Library, 2012), 35. Reprinted by permission of the authors.
5. Darcey Steinke, *Flash Count Diary: Menopause and the Vindication of Natural Life* (New York: Farrar, Straus and Giroux, 2019), 190.

Notes

Chapter 10

1. "WHO Coronavirus (COVID-19) Dashboard," World Health Organization, updated March 3, 2021, https://covid19.who.int.

2. Gregg Braden, *Fractal Time: The Secret of 2012 and a New World Age* (New York: Hay House, 2009), 62.

BIBLIOGRAPHY

Acton, William. *The Functions and Disorders of the Reproductive Organs in Childhood, Youth, Adult Age, and Advanced Life: Considered in Their Physiological, Social, and Moral Relations.* 3rd ed. London: Churchill, 1862.

"Adrenal Fatigue Diet." Women's Health Network. December 22, 2020. https://www.womenshealthnetwork.com/adrenal-fatigue-and-stress/the-adrenal-fatigue-diet.

Agur, Anne M. R., and Arthur F. Dalley. *Grant's Atlas of Anatomy.* 13th ed. Baltimore, MD: Lippincott Williams & Wilkins, 2013.

Alinat, Carissa. *The Menopause Switch: Disrupt Aging & Live Your Best Life Past Midlife.* Dunedin, FL: Origin Weightloss LLC, 2020.

Anderson, Gillian, and Jennifer Nadel. "The Truth Is Out There (About Menopause)." *Lenny Letter*, March 7, 2017. https://www.lennyletter.com/story/the-truth-is-out-there-about-menopause.

Arrien, Angeles. *The Second Half of Life: Opening the Eight Gates of Wisdom.* Boulder, CO: Sounds True, 2005.

Bertrand, Azra, and Seren Bertrand. *Womb Awakening: Initiatory Wisdom from the Creatrix of All Life.* Rochester, VT: Bear & Company, 2017.

Braden, Gregg. Fractal Time: *The Secret of 2012 and a New World Age.* New York: Hay House, 2009.

Brooks, Garth. "Standing Outside the Fire." Cowritten by Jenny Yates. December 13, 1993. Capitol, LP vinyl.

Brown, Brené. *Daring Greatly: How the Courage to be Vulnerable Transforms the Way We Live, Love, Parent, and Lead.* New York: Avery, 2012.

Bush, Zach. "Nutrition: The Gut Brain Axis and Human Performance." December 3, 2020. *Global Health Education Podcast.* Podcast, audio, 1:38:58. https://zachbushmd.com/knowledge-nutrition/?mc_cid=edc56b31f1&mc_eid=68006fb264.

Carlson, Kristine. *From Heartbreak to Wholeness: The Hero's Journey to Joy*. New York: St. Martin's Press, 2018.

Carstensen, Laura. *A Long Bright Future: An Action Plan for a Lifetime of Happiness, Health, and Financial Security*. New York: Public Affairs, 2011.

Carter, Niyaso. *Tantra: Sex for the Soul—Easy Steps to More Intimacy, Passion, Pleasure & Love*. Paia, HI: Sacred Loving Institute, 2016. Audiobook read by the author, 6:13:00.

Cartwright, Mark. "The Pillow Book." *World History Encyclopedia*. Updated April 20, 2017. https://www.ancient.eu/the_pillow_book.

Chödrön, Pema. *When Things Fall Apart: Heart Advice for Difficult Times*. Boulder, CO: Shambhala Publications, 1997.

Chopich, Erika J., and Margaret Paul. *Healing Your Aloneness: Finding Love and Wholeness through Your Inner Child*. San Francisco: Harper San Francisco, 1990.

Dodson, Betty. *Sex for One: The Joy of Selfloving*. New York: Three Rivers Press, 1996.

Doyle, Glennon. *Untamed*. New York: Dial Press, 2020.

Eiseley, Loren. *The Unexpected Universe*. New York: Harcourt Brace & Company, 1972.

Ensler, Eve. *The Vagina Monologues*. New York: Villard Books, 2001.

"Essential Oils for Sleep." American Sleep Association. Accessed August 17, 2020. https://www.sleepassociation.org/sleep-treatments/essential-oils-for-sleep.

Estés, Clarissa Pinkola. *The Late Bloomer: Myths & Stories of the Wise Woman Archetype*. Louisville, CO: Sounds True, 2012. Audiobook read by the author, 7:50:00.

Estes, Clarissa Pinkola. *Women Who Run with the Wolves: Myths and Stories of the Wild Woman Archetype*. New York: Ballantine Books, 1996.

"Exploring Deborah Tannen's Sex, Lies, and Conversation." PhD diss. Updated January 26, 2021. https://phdessay.com/exploring-deborah-tannens-sex-lies-and-conversation.

Bibliography

Faubion, Stephanie S. *The Mayo Clinic Menopause Solution: A Doctor's Guide to Relieving Hot Flashes, Enjoying Better Sex, Sleeping Well, Controlling Your Weight, and Being Happy.* New York: Time Inc. Books, 2017.

Fishman, Loren, and Ellen Saltonstall. *Yoga for Osteoporosis: The Complete Guide.* New York: W. W. Norton Company, 2010.

Gaines, Edwene. *The Four Spiritual Laws of Prosperity: A Simple Guide to Unlimited Abundance.* Emmaus, PA: Rodale Books, 2005.

Gibran, Kahlil. *Kahlil Gibran: The Collected Works.* New York: Alfred A. Knopf, 2007.

Gross, Terry, and Mary Pipher. "Aging Offers Women Enormous Possibilities for Growth." February 27, 2019. Fresh Air. Produced by WHYY. Podcast, MP3, 0:19:55. https://www.npr.org/2019/02/27/698535498/aging-offers-women-enormous-possibilities-for-growth-says-author.

Herbenick, Debby et al., "Women's Experiences with Genital Touching, Sexual Pleasure, and Orgasm: Results from a U.S. Probability Sample of Women Ages 18 to 94." *Journal of Sex and Marital Therapy* 44 (2018): 201–12. https://doi.org/10.1080/0092623X.2017.1346530.

Hillesum, Etty. *An Interrupted Life and Letters from Westerbork.* New York: Henry Holt, 1996.

Holt-Lunstad, Julianne, et al. "Loneliness and Social Isolation as Risk Factors for Mortality." *Perspectives on Psychological Science* 10, no. 2 (2015): 227–37. https://doi.org/10.1177/1745691614568352.

Hornaday, William T. *The Extermination of the American Bison 1886–87.* Washington, DC: Government Printing Office, 1889.

Huber, Cheri. *There Is Nothing Wrong with You: Going Beyond Self-Hate.* Chicago: Keep It Simple Books, 2001.

Kahn, Matt. "The Pain of Loss." *All for Love.* YouTube video, 1:33:18. June 12, 2018. https://www.youtube.com/watch?v=0kXVcGGwqwA.

Bibliography

Katie, Byron, and Stephen Mitchell. *Loving What Is: Four Questions That Can Change Your Life.* New York: Crown Archetype, 2002.

LaPorte, Danielle. *The Desire Map: A Guide to Creating Goals with Soul.* Boulder, CO: Sounds True, 2014.

Larsen, Gail. *Transformational Speaking: If You Want to Change the World, Tell a Better Story.* Berkeley, CA: Celestial Arts, 2007.

Lipton, Bruce. *The Biology of Belief: Unleashing the Power of Consciousness, Matter & Miracles.* New York: Hay House, 2016.

Loehr, Anne. "How Menopause Silently Affects 27 Million Women at Work Every Day." Fast Company. Updated February 17, 2016. https://www.fastcompany.com/3056703/how-menopause-silently-affects-27-million-women-at-work-every-day.

Macy, Joanna, and Chris Johnstone. *Active Hope: How to Face the Mess We're in without Going Crazy.* Novato, CA: New World Library, 2012.

Macy, Joanna, and Molly Young Brown. *Coming Back to Life: The Updated Guide to the Work That Reconnects.* Gabriola Island, BC: New Society Publishers, 2014.

Macy, Joanna, and Sam Mowe. "The Work That Reconnects." *Tricycle.* Spring, 2015. https://tricycle.org/magazine/work-reconnects.

Marcus, Aubrey. "Ecstasy in Life and Death with Dr. Zach Bush, MD." December 2, 2020. *Aubrey Marcus Podcast #285.* Podcast, audio, 1:57:00. https://www.aubreymarcus.com/blogs/aubrey-marcus-podcast/ecstasy-in-life-and-death-with-dr-zach-bush-md-amp-285.

"Menopause 101: A Primer for the Perimenopausal." North American Menopause Society. Accessed January 21, 2020. http://www.menopause.org/for-women/menopauseflashes/menopause-symptoms-and-treatments/menopause-101-a-primer-for-the-perimenopausal.

Nagoski, Emily. *Come As You Are: The Surprising New Science That Will Transform Your Sex Life.* New York: Simon & Schuster, 2015.

Bibliography

Newman, Gemma. *The Plant Power Doctor: A Simple Prescription for a Healthier You*. London: Ebury Press, 2021.

Ni, Maoshing. *Second Spring: Dr. Mao's Hundreds of Natural Secrets for Women to Revitalize and Regenerate at Any Age*. New York: Atria, 2009.

Northrup, Christiane. *The Wisdom of Menopause: Creating Physical and Emotional Health and Healing*. 5th ed. New York: Bantam, 2020.

Nuzzo, Regina. "The Science of Orgasm." *Los Angeles Times*, September 15, 2014. https://www.latimes.com/health/la-he-orgasm11feb11-story.html.

Pailet, Xanet. *Living an Orgasmic Life: Heal Yourself and Awaken Your Pleasure*. Miami, FL: Mango, 2018.

Palsdottir, Hrefna. "Nine Benefits of Maca Root and Potential Side Effects." *Healthline*. Updated October 30, 2016. https://www.healthline.com/nutrition/benefits-of-maca-root.

Parton, Dolly. *PMS Blues*. September 27, 1994. Columbia, LP vinyl.

Pelz, Mindy. *The Menopause Reset: Get Rid of Your Symptoms and Feel Like Your Younger Self Again*. Las Vegas, NV: Lifestyle Entrepreneurs Press, 2020.

Perel, Esther. *Mating in Captivity: Unlocking Erotic Intelligence*. New York: Harper Paperbacks, 2017.

Pipher, Mary. *Women Rowing North: Navigating Life's Currents and Flourishing as We Age*. New York: Bloomsbury, 2019.

Pope, Alexandra, and Sjanie Hugo Wurlitzer. *Wild Power: Discover the Magic of Your Menstrual Cycle and Awaken the Feminine Path to Power*. London: Hay House UK, 2017.

Rice, Sandra. *The Estrogen Question: Know Before You Say "No" to HRT*. Bellevue, WA: Rice-Nizlek Associates, 2019.

Skipper, Cathy. *The Alchemy of Menopause: The Journey of Stepping into Our Power and Becoming Who We Truly Are*. Scott's Valley, CA: CreateSpace, 2020.

Steinke, Darcey. *Flash Count Diary: Menopause and the Vindication of Natural Life*. New York: Farrar, Straus and Giroux, 2019.

Bibliography

Tannen, Deborah. *You Just Don't Understand: Women and Men in Conversation.* New York: William Morrow, 2006.

Taylor, S .E., et al. "Biobehavioral Responses to Stress in Females: Tend-and-Befriend, Not Fight-or-Flight." *Psychological Review* 107, no. 3 (2000): 411–29. https://doi.org/10.1037/0033-295X.107.3.411.

Velez, Adriana. "Menopause Is Different for Women of Color." Endocrine Web. Updated May 18, 2020. https://www.endocrineweb.com/menopause-different-women-color.

Villines, Zawn. "What to Know about Vaginal Lubrication." *Medical News Today,* September 25, 2019. https://www.medicalnewstoday.com/articles/326450.

von Fürstenberg, Diane. *The Woman I Wanted to Be.* New York: Simon & Schuster, 2014.

Weil, Andrew. *Healthy Aging: A Lifelong Guide to Your Well-Being.* New York: Knopf, 2005.

Weiser, Kathy. "The Cherokee Trail of Tears." *Legends of America.* Updated May 2020. https://www.legendsofamerica.com/na-trailtears.

William, Anthony. *Medical Medium Life-Changing Foods: Save Yourself and the Ones You Love with the Hidden Healing Powers of Fruits & Vegetables.* Carlsbad, CA: Hay House, 2016.

Wilson, Robert. *Feminine Forever.* New York: M. Evans and Company, 1966.

"The Witch Trials." *Western Civilization.* Course content for Lumen Learning. Accessed November 2, 2019. https://courses.lumenlearning.com/suny-hccc-worldhistory/chapter/the-witch-trials.

World Health Organization. "WHO Coronavirus (COVID-19) Dashboard." Updated March 3, 2021. https://covid19.who.int.

Wright, Hillary, and Elizabeth M. Ward. *The Menopause Diet Plan: A Natural Guide to Managing Hormones, Health, and Happiness.* Emmaus, PA: Rodale Books, 2020.

Zawalick, Zoe. *The Secret Life of Hormones: Finding Hormone Balance for a Better Life.* Independently published, 2020.

ABOUT THE AUTHOR

Lee Sumner Irwin is a spiritual teacher and intuitive guide specializing in women's transformation. Founder of the Radiant Wise Woman pro-age movement, she helps women in their forties and beyond give birth to their unique gifts and creative energy—a passion that has earned her the epithet "midwife for midlife." With thirty years of education and experience as a professional coach, occupational therapist, and international retreat leader, she has worked with hundreds of women worldwide in their quest to become more sexually alive and emotionally free.

Lee enjoys life with her spouse at the confluence of rivers and mountains in Birmingham, Alabama, where she can often be found stargazing with her grandchildren or drumming in a forest. This is her first book.

Made in the USA
Las Vegas, NV
22 March 2022